AMPUTATED SOULS

The Psychiatric Assault on Liberty
1935–2011

ANTHONY JAMES

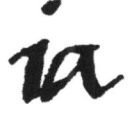

imprint-academic.com

Copyright © Anthony James, 2013

The moral rights of the author have been asserted.
No part of this publication may be reproduced in any form
without permission, except for the quotation of brief passages
in criticism and discussion.

Published in the UK by
Imprint Academic, PO Box 200, Exeter EX5 5YX, UK

Distributed in the USA by
Ingram Book Company,
One Ingram Blvd., La Vergne, TN 37086, USA

ISBN 9781845404505

A CIP catalogue record for this book is available from the
British Library and US Library of Congress

This book is dedicated to the millions of victims who have been denied a voice

'Further, I took with me certain simple criteria with which to measure the life of the underworld. That which made for more life, for physical and spiritual health, was good; that which made for less life, which hurt, and dwarfed, and distorted life, was bad.'

—Jack London

The names of individuals known to me personally have been changed in this book, and information that could point to their identities has been omitted. On the other hand, the reader will find that a very large part of the information used in this book has been drawn from the technical literature of psychiatry and mental health nursing.

Contents

Introduction: 'Eyeless in Gaza'	1
Chapter One: 'History to the Defeated'	8
Chapter Two: The Show Takes to the Road	31
Chapter Three: The Chemical Straitjacket	48
Chapter Four: Suitable Cases for Study: Psychiatry in Literature and Film	69
Chapter Five: Informed Consent	105
Chapter Six: The Situation Today	113
Chapter Seven: Freedom, Rights and Rape	123

Introduction
'Eyeless in Gaza'

In the 1980s, when I worked in a drug advice unit based in the community, it had become painfully obvious that the medical profession was capable of making mistakes on a huge scale. Millions of people across the developed world had been prescribed benzodiazepine tranquillisers like diazepam (Valium) and lorazepam, and led to believe that these drugs could be taken, even at high doses, for months or years, and then withdrawn from one day to the next without any problems. In fact, benzodiazepines are highly addictive, and a huge number of people worldwide (including myself in my twenties) found themselves addicted and in need of support for a prolonged period, usually several months, in order to free themselves from this dependency.

Books on pharmacology began to describe the consequences of the long-term use of tranquillisers quite unequivocally: 'All of the minor tranquillisers are, nevertheless, addictive [...] They can all lead to compulsive use and physical dependence. Withdrawal can cause psychotic behaviour, convulsions and coma, and has even been fatal.'[1] The prevailing wisdom among doctors, according to which only 'neurotic' or 'unstable' or 'maladjusted' individuals got themselves hooked on tranquillisers, quietly crept out by the back door, quite scared and unnerved by the outburst of anger among ordinary people and in the media and the mushrooming of self-help groups in which

---

[1] Richard B. Fisher and George A. Christie, *A Dictionary of Drugs*, revised edition, London, 1982.

people shared experiences of their involuntary addiction and gave each other support.

A book called *I'm Dancing as Fast as I Can*, in which Barbara Gordon (a respected American television producer) told the story of her unwitting addiction to diazepam and the terrifying symptoms of abruptly giving it up, was eagerly read by many middle-aged ladies who had been prescribed benzodiazepines, and then patronised and misinformed for decades.[2]

I was sent on a number of training courses as part of my work in the drug advice unit, and found myself—I think the year was 1985—among an endearingly diverse group of people, very typical of the eighties, at a conference centre just outside a village in the countryside of south-western England. Black Born-Again Christians, militant Marxists from African and Asian families, serious middle-class members of the Socialist Workers Party, genteel English ladies, misfits like myself, lesbian feminists and heterosexual feminists, and an ex-navvy from Belfast who had turned to social work, all of us involved in community work projects, came together for training on a course called 'Coping with the Mentally Ill', paid for by the organisations for which we worked.

We were asked a question by one of the tutors of the course, a psychiatric social worker, during one of the sessions: 'Well, what kind of treatment for mental illness do *you* find acceptable and what treatment do you find unacceptable?' A thoughtful, if awkward, silence followed.

'I think that any treatment that threatens the integrity of the individual is unacceptable', I suggested, noticing a moment later that the warmest approval for my words came from the lesbian feminists. The discussion went on for a long time until the same tutor made a remark that silenced us again.

'In the late 1940s and 1950s, psychiatric hospitals were handing out lobotomies as readily as general hospitals were doing tonsillectomies.'

---

[2] Barbara Gordon, *I'm Dancing as Fast as I Can*, London, 1980.

Introduction: 'Eyeless in Gaza'

I had, of course, done my best to study mental illness and psychiatric practice since working for the drug advice unit, dealing, as I did, almost exclusively with people who had problems with drugs prescribed for anxiety disorders and depression. I knew something about the brain operation known as a lobotomy and its history and development, as well as its widespread use in the past. I had visited some of those who came to us for advice when they were admitted to psychiatric hospitals, and there I had noticed middle-aged or elderly men—who tend to suffer from baldness—with quite striking scars at the top of the forehead, twin indentations on either side, evenly spaced. However, on that day on a training course, I began to wonder how much I did know.

The terms lobotomy, frontal lobotomy, pre-frontal lobotomy, leucotomy—occasionally spelt 'leukotomy'—do not have precisely the same meaning, as we shall see later, but in practice they are used fairly interchangeably to refer to an irreversible surgical operation on the brain that profoundly affects personality. I shall try to be clear about the subject of this book from the very beginning, and in doing so I must now quote some very basic definitions. In 1985, I had already encountered this description of lobotomy by Peter Wingate in the 1976 edition of *The Penguin Medical Encyclopedia*:

> A surgical operation devised in 1935 by Egas Moniz (1874–1955), a Portuguese neurosurgeon, for the relief of certain severe and progressive mental disturbances. The nerve cells of the pre-frontal lobes at the very front of the brain are disconnected from the rest of the brain by cutting the underlying fibres. [...] Since brain tissue cannot heal, the operation is irrevocable. People who have had it have altered personalities: they tend to be irresponsible. But most of us would rather be carefree than suicidal.[3]

This author, Peter Wingate, qualified as a doctor and practised for many years in colonial Africa, and we can, perhaps, put his positive attitude to lobotomy into perspective by looking at his

---

[3] Peter Wingate, *The Penguin Medical Encyclopedia*, Harmondsworth, 1976.

remarks on another subject in the same encyclopedia. Under the heading 'homosexuality', we find:

> Attempts to treat homosexuality often fail. Unless the subject strongly wishes to change, they are bound to fail [...] homosexuality is a handicap, and many of those affected never really come to terms with it. With young subjects (say, within 10 or 12 years of puberty) there is at least some chance that *behaviour therapy* may succeed [...] Some German surgeons have performed minor operations on the brain to suppress certain reflex centres thought to govern homosexual behaviour, again in the hope of keeping persistent offenders out of prison. They claim that some of their patients are not only cured of their criminal tendencies but have become heterosexual. For the present, this cannot be regarded as more than an interesting experiment.

Interesting, indeed! I would suggest that the most interesting aspect of this doctor's comments is not the way in which readers in the first decades of the twenty-first century might view them, but rather the fact that they could appear *in a standard medical text as late as 1976*. The way in which Dr Wingate effortlessly conflates homosexuality, paedophilia, and rape in the somewhat abridged passage quoted above is even more interesting (a 'persistent offender' would only be in prison for committing one of these crimes, not simply because of his sexual preferences).

The history of lobotomy as a medical procedure — but most of all as a social phenomenon — reveals, I believe, many, many more examples of individuals being defined as 'sick' or 'in need of treatment' simply because society did not like their choice of bed partners, or because society simply found *their gender* (the female gender without exception in this context) threatening in itself, or because they were regarded as troublemakers, or as undesirable members of the community who should be controlled.

Twelve years after that sunlit Gloucestershire morning in summer, I stood in Auschwitz, in which a very negative view of homosexuality had also prevailed, and in which another 'German surgeon', Dr Joseph Mengele, had also performed 'interesting experiments'. I had gone to Auschwitz partly because of my lifelong interest in the work of the scientist and philosopher Dr Jacob Bronowski (1908–1974), who had lost many members of his family in the death camp. It is Bronowski who provides the second very basic definition of lobotomy:

> We do not know exactly what the frontal lobes may do. We do not know anything very exactly [...] They make behaviour into patterns. They take the past and pattern it so that it is usable for the future. They organise behaviour. If you do an operation, as people foolishly did, twenty or thirty years ago, in which you cut off the frontal lobes from the rest of the brain, you get an extremely happy animal that you still call a man, but which is quite incapable of making any future-directed decision.[4]

Bronowski gives us the voice of science, although he was not a doctor, and we might criticise him for the words 'extremely happy', and for the excessively mild word 'foolishly'.

The writings of Wingate and Bronowski were two of the many authorities that contributed to my knowledge of lobotomy—such as it was—in the summer of 1985. Many people at that time recalled Ken Kesey's novel *One Flew Over the Cuckoo's Nest* (1962), given a massive new readership by the 1975 film of the same name, directed by Milos Forman.[5]

In the novel and in the film McMurphy, the central character, is given a lobotomy simply because he rebels against a suffocating and oppressive system. Lobotomy and electric shock therapy are held up as the ultimate terror and deterrent by that system—a microcosm of society in general—combining insidiously with a still more powerful mechanism of control, namely the fear and apathy of the patients/citizens. Here, of course, we come to the crucial and cruel question. What is lobotomy—medically, morally, and socially—*why* was it used in the past, and *why* is it used today?

Perhaps it was a responsibly developed clinical procedure that was used only as a last resort to relieve the suffering of

---

[4] Jacob Bronowski, *Journey Round a Twentieth Century Skull* (the last broadcasts), *The Listener*, May 15–July 3 1975.
[5] Ken Kesey, *One Flew Over the Cuckoo's Nest*, London, 1962.

people who could not be expected to respond to any other treatment. If so, we would expect the operation to have been performed on a small number of men and women, and we would regard those men and women in the same way as we regard the victims of other severe and incurable illnesses who have received drastic surgery in a desperate attempt to help them. We may even have to face a still more unpleasant fact. Lobotomy, it is claimed, was performed to relieve otherwise incurable mental illness, and so it may have been used to control the behaviour of highly dangerous people who would otherwise have been imprisoned for the rest of their natural lives. On the other hand, if we find that this 'irreversible' and 'irrevocable' operation was performed upon a large number of patients, if we find that men and women had their brains and personalities changed or reduced only because they suffered from the unhappiness, uneasiness, stress, and inadequacy that afflicts all human beings, then we are confronted by something very different, something very disturbing. And worse still, we may find that this operation was used upon women and men like ourselves because their sexual habits or even their political beliefs were disliked by the powerful individuals who manage our affairs.

I shall look at the history, development and use of lobotomy, and of electro-convulsive therapy or ECT, in this book, drawing upon evidence that can be regarded as reliable beyond reasonable doubt, as well as upon the more subjective account of this distressing subject that can be drawn from both creative and medical literature. History is surely a futile activity if it does not make connections and draw conclusions: connections will be made and conclusions drawn as often as possible in this book.

I believe that the widespread use of a brain operation that changes or reduces the personality of human beings, as well as the motives for performing such an operation, tell us a great deal about a society that accepts this procedure and these motives. The actions of Joseph Mengele in performing agonising and frequently fatal experiments upon prisoners in Auschwitz, including children and physically handicapped persons, were entirely consistent with Nazi anti-values. Any society that tolerates the use of radical, invasive, and life-changing surgery upon selected individuals, undertaken gratuitously or upon flimsy empirical evidence, must question the very values that it claims to embrace.

We shall return to what might be called common wisdom and the popular consciousness a little further on, bearing in mind that this wisdom and consciousness may or may not accord with demonstrable fact. Popular wisdom conceives of lobotomy very much as it is portrayed in *One Flew Over the Cuckoo's Nest*—the worst of all fates, a kind of execution without death, a modern manifestation of the castration of Abelard after his passionate relationship with Heloise, and of the blinding of Samson, kept alive to be mocked, in Milton's words 'Eyeless in Gaza, at the mill, with slaves'.

If the actions of actual medical practitioners can be shown to justify this popular repugnance and fear, so that we find those who promoted and carried out lobotomies to be guilty of an enormous betrayal of trust, then our society also stands condemned. We would have to conclude that the community, whatever deep and instinctive fears it harboured, had to some extent acquiesced in the intolerable. It is worth recording the ironic fact that Auschwitz is in the town of Oswiecim in Poland, south of Krakow. We might say that Joseph Conrad, the son of a Polish nobleman and political prisoner, spending part of his childhood in Krakow near to the site upon which Auschwitz was later established, was to foresee the hateful *spirit* of Nazism in his work, although he could not have foreseen its actuality. Conrad became one of the greatest novelists in English, and is irrevocably associated with the words 'heart of darkness', too often quoted but still richly suggestive. It is not, perhaps, too much of an exaggeration to say that an exploration of the whole issue of lobotomy is one of the paths into the heart of darkness at the centre of our own society.

Chapter One

'History to the Defeated'

The story of Salvatore, an American citizen of Italian descent, is told by Dr Judith Rapoport in her fairly humane and constructive book on OCD, Obsessive-Compulsive Disorder.[1] Salvatore was once a happy husband and father, a valued workman and a churchgoer, and then he fell ill with OCD and developed the irresistible compulsion to pick up rubbish in the streets and hoard it in bags in his home in ever increasing quantities, making his relationship with his wife impossible. He was hospitalized in the 1940s and given a prefrontal lobotomy. Salvatore's compulsions ceased after the lobotomy, however, he developed other behaviour, such as pinching strange young women and urinating in the street, that was found unacceptable, and so he was never allowed to leave hospital.

Lobotomies had been performed for about a decade by the time the operation was given to Salvatore, and so the effects, including post-lobotomy behaviour such as his, were well known. I believe that it is necessary for the student of history, like the student of philosophy, to ask simple-minded and even naïve questions. For instance, why would urinating in the street and molesting young women and spending life in a mental hospital be seen as in any way preferable to collecting and hoarding bits of rubbish, even if that compulsion did destroy Salvatore's marriage? Salvatore still lost his family and his

---

[1] Dr Judith L. Rapoport, *The Boy Who Couldn't Stop Washing*, London, 1990.

occupation. After all, the lobotomy was irreversible, whereas common sense, our experiences in life, and the entire history of medicine all demonstrate that many conditions improve or disappear with time, especially if prolonged care and attention are given to the sufferer. Salvatore might have remained a free citizen, albeit a somewhat lonely, tortured, and eccentric one, and he might have salvaged some kind of relationship with his wife, or made a life with some woman who was as strange and eccentric as himself.

In her book, published in 1990, Dr Rapoport states: 'In the most severe cases of OCD, psychosurgery was used regularly until the 1950s [...] I have yet to send a patient for such treatment.' We can only wonder whether the word *yet* was disturbing to her readers and her patients, four decades after Salvatore's treatment and twenty-eight years after the publication of *One Flew Over the Cuckoo's Nest*.

Five years later, in 1995, and a full decade after the experiences and discussions I quoted in my introduction, we still read the following in the thirty-eighth edition of *Black's Medical Dictionary*: 'Patients are only considered for psychosurgery when they have failed to respond to routine therapies. One contra-indication is marked histrionic or anti-social personality.'[2] This standard reference work advised its readers that 'a favourable response' to psychosurgery might be expected in cases of 'chronic obsessional neuroses, anxiety states and severe chronic depression'.

Psychosurgery has required the consent of the patient under the 1983 and 2007 Mental Health Acts in England and Wales, although electro-convulsive therapy, ECT, also commonly known as electric shock treatment, can be given against a person's will in certain circumstances under the same Acts. The notion of 'informed consent' is a difficult one, morally and practically, and I shall return to it later.

Professor Colin Blakemore devotes a good deal of space to the subject of lobotomy/leucotomy and ECT in the 1976 BBC Reith

---

[2] G. Macpherson, editor, *Black's Medical Dictionary*, London, 1995.

Lectures, which formed the basis of his book *Mechanics of the Mind*, and in this chapter I shall be quoting and drawing upon the texts of the lectures published in the journal *The Listener*.[3]

Blakemore became Professor of Physiology at Oxford University after eleven years in the Department of Physiology at Cambridge, and has been Chief Executive of the Medical Research Council since 2003. And although he has sometimes been a controversial figure, I shall concentrate upon his social and historical analysis of some issues, ignoring the particular controversies that his work has aroused that do not concern us here.

Many people quite reasonably fear that medical manipulation of the brain might be used by power-hungry politicians in order to tighten their control over society, but in fact, the sheer time, expense, and technical difficulty involved in such large-scale behaviour control would make it impractical. However, Professor Blakemore argues that the use of psychosurgery upon the mentally ill is 'certainly the closest that we come to the horror of socially-applied control of the brain, and it illustrates both the inadequate restraints on the treatment of the mentally sick and the poor theoretical basis for that therapy [...] that would be considered inadequate in all other areas of medicine'.

The story of modern psychosurgery begins with a research report delivered by C. Jacobsen and J.F. Fulton at a conference of neurologists held in London in 1935. The researchers described their experiments upon the abilities of two chimpanzees to remember where small portions of food were hidden, and they reported that one of the chimpanzees, called Becky, became angry and anxious when she failed to find the food, flying into a rage and refusing to perform. Fulton and Jacobsen performed an operation on Becky in which they cut out part of the frontal lobes of the cerebral hemispheres of her brain. They reported that the result of this operation was that Becky no longer became emotional when she failed to find the hidden

---

[3] Colin Blakemore, The 1976 BBC Reith Lectures, *The Listener*, especially December 16 1976. See also Colin Blakemore, *Mechanics of the Mind*, Cambridge, 1977.

food during experiments. Egas Moniz (1874–1955), a Portuguese neurosurgeon and Professor of Medicine at Lisbon University, rose to his feet after the lecture to ask the following question: 'If frontal lobe removal prevents the development of experimental neuroses in animals and eliminates frustration behaviour, why would it not be feasible to relieve anxiety states in man by surgical means?'

Moniz, it must be pointed out, had made a serious contribution to medicine in the 1930s by developing the imaging of living brain tissue by angiography (the injection of substances opaque to X-rays into the cerebral arteries), which allowed neurosurgeons to find the precise location of brain tumours. He had probably expected to receive the Nobel Prize for this work, and his invention the prefrontal leucotomy operation may well have been driven partly by personal ambition, or 'frustration behaviour' as he called it. Moniz returned to Portugal and began to perform leucotomies on psychiatric patients, in association with a surgeon named Almeida Lima.

F.A. Whitlock, a Professor of Psychiatry in the University of Queensland, Australia, writing in 1987, rather laconically assesses the first twenty patients who were given leucotomies by Moniz: 'Although the operation was crude, of the first twenty cases seven recovered and seven improved.'[4] And yet, as Colin Blakemore reminds us in the 1976 Reith Lectures, the definition of recovery and improvement can be highly subjective: 'the effectiveness of these operations was evaluated by the very surgeons who had invested their careers in psychosurgery: failure was not easy to accept.'

Blakemore also points out the sheer scale of the phenomenon that had originated in that conference of neurologists in London in 1935: 'by 1950 some 20,000 people around the world, including prisoners and children, had been treated this way. And all of this stemmed from an almost anecdotal observation on a single, nervous chimpanzee.' In Britain leucotomy was carried out on 10,365 psychiatric patients between 1942 and

---

[4] F.A. Whitlock, 'Psychosurgery', in *The Oxford Companion to the Mind*, edited by Richard L. Gregory, Oxford, 1987.

1954.⁵ Whitlock tells us, in the same article in 1987, that of these patients 'only 3 per cent showed undesirable side-effects and that more than 40 per cent had been ill for at least six years. The operation was performed in only a few centres, a fact which seems to imply that, regardless of its alleged usefulness, attitudes opposing it were strongly held by medical staff in many hospitals.' It should be added that the figure of 10,365 patients subjected to leucotomy is derived only from England and Wales.

Professor Richard P. Bentall, a clinical psychologist, described an elderly woman he met in the North Wales Hospital, near the town of Denbigh, when he was a student in the 1970s: '[She] kept insisting that "Peter Pickering has plucked my brain", a delusion which became more intelligible when inspection of her case notes revealed that she had been given a prefrontal leucotomy.' This operation had been carried out under a local anaesthetic only, so that the woman became 'highly distressed' when the knife entered her brain.

Bentall also describes the fate of Egas Moniz himself, who eventually got his Nobel Prize in 1949, but did not enjoy his fame for as long as he may have anticipated. The death of Moniz was 'one of the more ironical twists in the history of psychiatry, Moniz was shot dead by a disgruntled leucotomy patient in 1955'.⁶ Perhaps the use of leucotomy would not have been so widespread if more of the patients who had been subjected to it had been capable of such strenuous and drastic action.

We must now look at another physical method used to treat mental illness that was also invented in the 1930s, three years after leucotomy. Professor Blakemore reminds us that electro-convulsive therapy, ECT, is 'based on even more obtuse and spurious theoretical justification'. Blakemore continues: 'The

---

5 G.C. Tooth and M.P. Newton, *Leucotomy in England and Wales, 1942–1954*, London, 1961. See also *The Oxford Companion to the Mind*, Oxford, 1987, above.
6 Richard P. Bentall, *Madness Explained: Psychosis and Human Nature*, London, 2003.

present-day use of convulsive therapy stems from a revival of the 18th-century opinion that maniacs were best treated by a very severe physical stress, and from the entirely erroneous view that epileptics are protected from schizophrenia by their natural convulsions.' If we are entitled to regard the history of leucotomy/lobotomy, beginning as it did with Moniz's excitement over the elimination of 'frustration behaviour' in 'a single, nervous chimpanzee', and continuing to his being shot in the spine by a lobotomised patient, as strange and morbid, then we may see the history of ECT as even more surreal. It began in a slaughterhouse.

Firstly, however, let us look at some precise definitions of this procedure: 'Applying a voltage, with surface electrodes on the head, across the brain. This is done under anaesthesia or muscle-relaxant, as it produces convulsions which can be dangerous. ECT is extensively used as a *convenient and quick* treatment for depression, though there is no theoretical basis to justify it' (*The Oxford Companion to the Mind*, Oxford, 1987). The italics are mine—the words, I believe, beg the question of *whose convenience* is referred to in this and in many, many similar descriptions of ECT.

There is disagreement about the nature of ECT and its consequences even among the authors of standard medical texts. Peter Wingate, whom I quoted in my introduction, tells us confidently: 'The convulsion had nothing to do with the efficacy of the treatment, and though the patient remembered nothing of it, there was a risk that it might cause him to injure himself while unconscious. Furthermore, the very idea of ECT alarms most patients.'[7]

Wingate makes no mention of the long-term effects of this treatment, but *Black's Medical Dictionary* (London, 1995) is quite unequivocal: 'Electrical shocks are administered by electrodes placed on the skull to induce seizures of the brain [...] Amnesia is often a side-effect of ECT.' Far from the seizure or convulsion being incidental, it is widely regarded by psychiatrists as being essential, it is 'a fit and then unconsciousness' that are deemed

---

[7] Peter Wingate, *The Penguin Medical Encyclopedia*, Harmondsworth, 1976.

beneficial, as Lisa Appignanesi reminds us in her recent history of the treatment of women by the psychiatric profession.[8]

We are, therefore, confronted by a radical intervention in the functioning of the brain of a woman or man that is not based on any clear understanding of the relationship between the 'treatment' and the condition that it is supposed to relieve. Further, this procedure artificially causes a fit or convulsion in the person subjected to it, and we must keep in mind the fact that seizures or convulsions have always been and continue to be regarded—except in the ECT room—as symptoms of a serious illness or disturbance of the nervous system or of injury to the brain. Finally, we see that in the eyes of those who uphold the 'efficacy' of ECT its virtues are quickness and convenience, and yet it is now recognised that many patients who are given this treatment must suffer other long-lasting disabilities in place of the condition that has allegedly been cured. These disturbing facts emerge from considering three widely read—though somewhat conflicting—works of reference that have been seen as irreproachable in their integrity, together with a highly celebrated historical work.

ECT was invented in Rome in 1938 by Dr Ugo Cerletti (1877–1963). Cerletti had studied medicine at Rome and Turin, and later in Paris and in Munich with Emil Kraepelin (1856–1926) who should be regarded—rather than Freud—as the founder of modern psychiatry. It was Kraepelin who devised the classification of psychotic illnesses by placing them in a small number of identifiable categories, a system that is still widely accepted today, although the growing body of evidence that contradicts this approach is enormous.[9]

Cerletti went on to become a professor at the University of Genoa, and then, in 1935 (the year of the conference at which Egas Moniz conceived of the surgical removal of the frontal

---

[8] Lisa Appignanesi, *Mad, Bad and Sad: A History of Women and the Mind Doctors from 1800 to the Present*, London, 2008.
[9] Richard P. Bentall, *Madness Explained: Psychosis and Human Nature*, London, 2003.

lobes) he took up the Chair of the Department of Mental and Neurological Diseases at the University of Rome La Sapienza.

Perhaps it is not entirely irrelevant to pause at this point and reflect upon the grandeur of the academic positions of men like Moniz and Cerletti, their prestige, power, and authority, and compare these to the powerlessness of the patients, usually despised and discarded by society, upon whom they imposed their discoveries. It is true, of course, that most scientists who have made discoveries—especially medical discoveries—have held professional and academic positions, but only in neurology and psychiatry have these discoveries been directed at changing the consciousness and personalities of men and women, frequently against their will.

Cerletti had already experimented with inducing repeated epileptic-like fits in dogs and other animals at Genoa and Rome. He visited a Rome slaughterhouse in 1938 (we can only wonder why—with a laboratory or laboratories at his disposal—he would do this, and it seems that his own account of this in an article on the subject, as far as can be judged so long afterwards, is unclear on this point).[10] He witnessed pigs being stunned by an electric shock to the head in the slaughterhouse, rendering them unconscious and shaken by convulsions, during which they were (apparently) unaware of being killed by stabbing with a knife. It was at this point that the idea of using electric shocks to the brains of people suffering from mental illnesses came to Cerletti.

ECT was first used on a human being by Cerletti soon afterwards, in April 1938, in an experiment in which he subjected a man regarded as a schizophrenic to an electric shock to the brain. The man shouted: 'Not a second one! It will kill me!' However, Cerletti went ahead anyway and gave the man another shock. The mental condition of this first patient to receive ECT was considered to be better after the electric shocks (here, it as well to recall Colin Blakemore's comment, 'the effectiveness of these operations was evaluated by the very

---

[10] Ugo Cerletti, 'L'Elettroshock' in *Rivista Sperimentale di Frenatria*, Volume 1, 209–310, 1940.

surgeons who had invested their careers in psychosurgery: failure was not easy to accept' — it is certain beyond reasonable doubt that this applied to ECT, and is still applicable today, more than seventy years later).

The use of artificially produced convulsions as a treatment for mental illness actually predated Cerletti and ECT, based as it was upon the notion that schizophrenia and epilepsy were antagonistic, but these methods involved the administration of Cardiozol, 'an unreliable camphor-based convulsive and [...] insulin therapy, which took an unpredictable period to build up the desired reaction of a convulsion or coma/sleep'.[11]

The acceptance and use of ECT quickly spread all over the world, although it seems initially to have been less popular in America. The procedure was welcomed more enthusiastically in Britain where the first use of ECT on patients was carried out by William Grey Walter (1910-1976) at the Burden Neurological Institute in Bristol using an ECT machine designed by Grey Walter, and yet, in the case of this physiologist, another 'ironical twist' in the history of psychiatry rears up: 'His highly productive work [...] was tragically halted in 1970 by a severe head injury from which he never fully recovered.'[12]

It is instructive to look at two sets of figures — referring to dates approximately four decades and approximately six decades after the invention of ECT and applying to the UK — in order to grasp the scale of Cerletti's legacy. In 1977 (the year after William Grey Walter died), it was estimated that psychiatrists in Britain gave as many as 100,000 ECT treatments and, as most patients are given about 10 or 12 treatments, this represents about 10,000 patients who underwent this procedure.[13] More recently, 2,800 patients in England received ECT treatment between January and March 1999, and 700 of these patients were detained under the Mental Health Act, with 59

---

[11] Lisa Appignanesi, *Mad, Bad and Sad: A History of Women and the Mind Doctors from 1800 to the Present*, London, 2008.

[12] Ray Cooper, 'William Grey Walter', in *The Oxford Companion to the Mind*, edited by Richard L. Gregory, Oxford, 1987.

[13] Julian Mounter, 'The right to refuse ECT', BBC 1 'Panorama' documentary, reprinted in *The Listener*, July 21 1977.

per cent of them being subjected to this treatment against their will, according to a massive textbook of 757 pages aimed at psychiatric nurses, to which I shall return further on.[14]

It is likely that ECT is used and regarded with favour by psychiatrists in Australia, Austria, Canada, Denmark, Germany, India, and The Netherlands, and it seems to be increasing in popularity among psychiatrists in Australia, Belgium, Greece, Hungary, India, Japan, Pakistan, and Russia. It may be worth noticing that among these countries only Denmark, Germany, The Netherlands, and possibly Belgium have a recent exemplary human rights record. ECT is still used widely in the USA, although in some American states it is banned by law.

Although psychiatrists—and even some of the patients who have been given ECT—argue in favour of its benefits today, the destructive and unwanted consequences of the treatment have been known from the very early days. Patients 'loathed and feared the passivity, the scrambling of memory, the zombie-like condition of those who came back from treatment'.[15] And in her autobiographical novel *The Bell Jar*, Sylvia Plath's heroine Esther Greenwood says of ECT: 'If anyone does that to me again I'll kill myself.'[16]

Another writer who experienced ECT and the mental havoc it caused was the American Nobel Prize winner Ernest Hemingway (1898–1961), who fell ill with depression in the last years before his death, although he was never to depict the experience in his writing—for good reason! It is claimed that ECT can lift the severe depression that makes the patient suicidal, but if so, it failed strikingly in the case of Hemingway, who shot himself, partly because of the effects of the treatment. His wife Mary described his condition while being subjected to ECT, at the Mayo Clinic in Rochester, Minnesota, in a telephone conversation with Hemingway's friend A.E. Hotchner: 'During the month of December, Ernest was given eleven treatments

---

[14] Phil Barker, editor, *Psychiatric and Mental Health Nursing*, 2nd edition, London, 2009.
[15] Lisa Appignanesi, *Mad, Bad and Sad: A History of Women and the Mind Doctors from 1800 to the Present*, London, 2008.
[16] Sylvia Plath, *The Bell Jar*, London, 1963.

with electric shock, technically referred to as ECT's. Mary told me about them, how terrible they were for Ernest and how he suffered, more psychologically than physically, from receiving them.'[17] In the same memoir, Hotchner records Hemingway's own bitter words about ECT: 'Well, what is the sense of ruining my head and erasing my memory, which is my capital, and putting me out of business? It was a brilliant cure but we lost the patient.' Hemingway was given more ECT in May 1961, and continued to state that he was now *incapable* of writing again, finally killing himself on July 2 that year.

From a literary point of view, Hemingway's work did, of course, decline in the last twenty years of his life, and it must be admitted that his depression and paranoid delusions might have pushed him into suicide anyway. On the other hand, without the degradation and humiliation of ECT and the memory loss that followed it, he might—with the right care and support and simply with the passage of time—have recovered and written some of his best work in old age. We will never know.

It was fortunate for Joseph Conrad, and for the world, that he lived and died before ECT was invented. Conrad was a greater writer than Hemingway, but he also suffered from pathological depression throughout the thirty years of his writing career—far longer than Hemingway—and he suffered a severe psychotic breakdown after completing *Under Western Eyes* in 1910. Would Conrad's dignity and ability to write also have been destroyed by Cerletti's invention if he had lived longer?

The destructive effects of ECT are acknowledged in medical literature today, although this was not done even a relatively short time ago. A standard text for psychiatric nurses published in 1985 comments on memory loss, but states cheerfully: 'This is the very thing which some patients worry about, if they happen to have heard about the loss of memory which follows ECT. In this case the doctor will assure the patient that loss of memory is only transitory and that there is no danger of important things

---

[17]   A.E. Hotchner, *Papa Hemingway, a Personal Memoir*, London, 1966.

being forgotten.'[18] The massive second edition of *Psychiatric and Mental Health Nursing* (2009) gives very different advice:

> Although ECT continues to have controversial status, there is a shift in the professional perspective which now maintains that service users must be fully informed of the potential risks and benefits of ECT before giving consent [...] The Royal College of Psychiatrists and NICE [National Institute for Health and Clinical Excellence] advise that the potential for cognitive impairment is highlighted during the consent process — the service user should be told that ECT may have serious and permanent effects on both memory and non-memory cognition.[19]

Or, we might say — bitterly, but not entirely facetiously — the 'service user' should be given a copy of *Papa Hemingway* to read, with the relevant pages marked! However, it is a tribute to the integrity of this textbook that it gives lengthy quotations from the testimony of patients who have undergone this procedure and found it destructive *as well as* quoting the words of those who have found ECT helpful. There are two statements by patients in the book that describe the experience of ECT as helpful and positive, and seven statements — remarkably similar to Hemingway's words recorded by Hotchner — that describe the treatment as having diminished ability, personality, and the quality of life.

Therefore, it is clear that ECT is a very serious procedure that may change the future life and the mental abilities or the personality of the person who undergoes it. How can subjecting a person to ECT against her/his wishes and without her/his consent ever be justified? No one suggests that the person suffering from severe cancer or arthritis should be forced to undergo radical surgery if she/he decides that prolonged pain or even death is preferable to that surgery. Similarly, a person may be suffering terrible anguish from severe depression or

---

[18] Annie Altschul and Margaret McGovern, *Psychiatric Nursing: A Concise Nursing Text*, 6th edition, London, 1985.

[19] Joy Bray, 'The nurse's role in the administration of electroconvulsive therapy', in *Psychiatric and Mental Health Nursing*, edited by Phil Barker, 2nd edition, London, 2009.

delusions or from hearing voices, and yet she/he decides that this suffering is preferable to ECT or psychosurgery. What possible moral justification can there be for overriding that choice? After all, my neighbour may believe—against all the evidence—that the Earth is flat and that Marilyn Monroe and Elvis Presley are still alive, but this does not mean that he cannot make a sensible and entirely valid decision to avoid cigarettes because they damage his lungs and to avoid mushrooms because they give him an upset stomach. And yet, even today, in certain circumstances, society removes independence of choice and respect for choice from those who are suffering from a mental illness—the very form of illness that is diagnosed very subjectively and is impossible to define clearly.

Larry Gostin of MIND, the National Association for Mental Health, described this situation in a 1976 documentary: 'People just tend to assume that someone who is mentally ill is not capable of making decisions, of understanding what is happening to him. But the royal commission that led up to the Mental Health Act was very clear on the point somebody who is mentally ill is not necessarily disabled, and it does not necessarily mean that they cannot say, "I don't want this treatment," or, "I would rather have something with fewer side-effects".'[20] And yet psychiatrists in our society—and so, to some extent, all of us—employ a Catch-22 when it comes to people who are mentally ill, a piece of 'mad' mental evasion that is eerily similar to the formula in Joseph Heller's great novel *Catch-22*. Heller's central character says he is mad and therefore unfit to go on further combat missions, but when he asks to go home he is told that he cannot be mad because no sane person would want to go on combat missions anyway.

In the very same 1976 documentary, Christopher Price, an MP who wanted to ban ECT (as some US states had already done) described this Catch-22 situation: 'I think it [ECT] is so dangerous that, in the long term, I would like to get rid of it completely. There is widespread abuse of the consent proced-

---

[20] Larry Gostin, MIND, in Julian Mounter, 'The right to refuse ECT', BBC 1 'Panorama' documentary, reprinted in *The Listener*, July 21 1977.

ures. If you say that you don't want this treatment, the doctors say, "Oh, yes, that is part of your illness, not wanting it." I think Parliament ought to pass some legislation to prevent these abuses.' Parliament did pass legislation, of course, in the form of the 1983 Mental Health Act, and more recently, the 2007 Mental Health Act, but the words of Larry Gostin of MIND — *'necessarily, necessarily'* — continue to haunt us. A mentally ill person is not *necessarily* disabled or unable to make a choice, but sometimes, it would seem, she/he is incapable of making a choice, and the wishes of others, such as psychiatrists and relatives, seeking a 'convenient and quick treatment' can be imposed on that person.

In February 2003, the case of K, a severely depressed woman aged forty-one, came before the High Court because she was granted a judicial review of the power of doctors to impose ECT on her. Stephen Field, K's barrister said: 'She doesn't want her head plugged into the mains and she is quite capable of giving cogent reasons for her decision.'[21]

I would suggest that however depressed, deluded, or hallucinated a person may be, her/his mental condition can *never* be taken as evidence that she/he is incapable of making a decision to reject a particular form of treatment. The notion that unnatural despair or delusions or suffering in *some* or in *many* areas of life invalidate the rejection of a specific course of action is completely mistaken.

Therefore, as reliable evidence of *incapacity* to make a choice can never be found, any society that claims to uphold the freedom, integrity, and autonomy of the individual must always assume that capacity exists, just as a citizen accused of a crime is innocent until proved guilty (with the difference that incapacity can never be proved but only asserted subjectively on the basis of inferences drawn by self-styled experts). I would also suggest that the rejection of a particular form of treatment should not have to be 'cogent' or articulate: a simple 'no' should suffice.

---

[21] Jeremy Laurance, Health Editor, 'Patient challenges electric shock therapy', *The Independent*, February 17 2003.

As morally and legally aware campaigners say of the crime of rape, 'No means no'. And yet the 1983 Mental Health Act amended by the 2007 Mental Health Act still allows a person to be forced to undergo ECT, although this has become more difficult to impose. Section 58 concerns treatment that requires consent *or* a second opinion for people detained under Sections of the Mental Health Act (commonly described as 'sectioned'), or for people defined as not able to give their informed consent. Under the 2007 Act not only an 'approved social worker', but also nurses, psychologists, and occupational therapists (approved mental health professionals) can make an application for a person to be detained, and so can a close relative.

Psychiatry at a Glance (2008), which is, despite its user-friendly and popular title, a textbook for the training of psychiatric professionals, sets out these details very concisely.[22] Treatments that fall under Section 58 are medication for a period of *more than* six months (but in the first six months the medication can be given without consent) and ECT.

If a person is seen as unable to understand the nature, purpose, and likely effects of the treatment and therefore cannot consent to it *or* is seen as able to understand but, being detained, refuses to consent to it, a doctor appointed by the Mental Health Act Commission is called in to give a second opinion, and must consult two people who have been 'professionally involved' in the person's treatment. If this doctor in his/her 'second opinion' agrees that the patient lacks the capacity to consent and ECT is in the patient's 'best interests' then it can be given against the person's will. Further, Section 62 allows for ECT to be given against a person's will on an emergency basis, in order to save the patient's life or prevent a 'serious deterioration' in the patient's condition. Obviously, ECT cannot save anyone's life. It is alleged that it can lift the severe depression that makes a patient suicidal or unwilling to eat, however, *Psychiatric and Mental Health Nursing* (2009) cautions us: 'Although one of the commonest reasons given for administering ECT is that it

---

[22] Cornelius Katona, Claudia Cooper and Mary Robertson, *Psychiatry at a Glance*, 4th edition, Oxford/Chichester, 2008.

prevents suicide, this assumption can be challenged [...] ECT does not necessarily prevent suicide in those with severe depression.' And this statement was published almost fifty years after the suicides of Ernest Hemingway and Sylvia Plath, who were both subjected to ECT!

The 2007 Act also provides for Supervised Community Treatment orders for detained patients when they return home, and if they fail to comply with these orders, 'they can be taken to a clinical setting and given treatment against their will'.[23] Interestingly, there was an increase in the number of people receiving ECT when detained under the Mental Health Act in 2006 compared to the years 1999 and 2002.[24]

I think that we can see the safeguards apparently included in the Mental Health Act in their true light if we consider that judgments such as 'unable to understand' treatment, or 'lacking the capacity' to give consent, or 'serious deterioration' in the patient's condition, or the patient's 'best interests', are all extremely subjective and conditioned by preconceived views of mentally ill people and by professional self-interest. As *Psychiatric and Mental Health Nursing* (2009) warns, even voluntary patients 'often experience the admission [i.e. to hospital] as coercive, with many subsequently attempting to leave, only to be compulsorily admitted to prevent them from doing so', while safeguards on the forcible use of ECT 'appear, at times, to be disregarded'. (I think that a word should be added about the politically correct language employed in this huge book, which is almost Orwellian, despite the considerable integrity of its content. The word 'patient' is repeatedly replaced by 'service user'. However, it is clear that people who are detained and compelled to undergo ECT are not using the Health Service, but rather being *used by* the Health Service.)

There are other issues that are relevant to liberty in this context, namely professional loyalty, collaboration, and connivance.

---

[23] Alan Nathan, 'Consent and the new mental health law', *The Pharmaceutical Journal*, Volume 280, June 21 2008.

[24] David Bickerton *et al.*, 'Trends in the administration of electroconvulsive therapy in England', *The Psychiatrist*, 33: 61–63, The Royal College of Psychiatrists, 2009.

Is the doctor appointed to give a second opinion in cases of refusal to consent to ECT more likely to support the decision of the patient or more likely to support the decision of fellow mental health professionals? The psychologist Richard P. Bentall, in his book *Madness Explained* (2003), quotes Walter Reich's explanation of the forcible psychiatric treatment of political dissidents in the Soviet Union by doctors who were acting in good faith: 'Those Soviet psychiatrists really *saw* the patients as schizophrenic [...] *[T]he system created a category, first on paper and then, with training, in the minds of Soviet psychiatrists* [...].' I do not think that we should assume that the same process is at all impossible in our own society today. In 1976, the Russian dissident Andrei Amalrik was even more explicit: 'those who are perhaps most sceptical about the whole question are a number of Western psychiatrists, because there is, of course, a certain etiquette among the members of the profession, and one psychiatrist will always have more faith in the words of another psychiatrist than of a patient.'[25]

Another Russian writer, Alexander Solzhenitsyn, also dealt with this moral issue while exposing Soviet oppression:

> To do evil a human being must first of all believe that what he's doing is good, or else that it's a well-considered act in conformity with natural law [...] Ideology [...] gives [...] the necessary steadfastness and determination. That is the social theory which helps to make his acts seem good instead of bad in his own and others' eyes, so that he won't hear reproaches and curses but will receive praise and honours.[26]

Psychiatry is certainly an 'ideology' (as all postmodernists will readily agree) and also a 'social theory'. We can see quite easily that psychiatry amounts to no more than these things if we reflect that mental illness and its treatment are *socially defined*. After all, some American states have banned ECT and the

---

[25] Andrei Amalrik in conversation with Michael Charlton, BBC 2 'Newsday', reprinted in *The Listener*, October 14 1976.
[26] Alexander Solzhenitsyn, *The Gulag Archipelago*, Volume 1, London, 1974.

powers of doctors over patients have waxed and waned in the UK with successive Mental Health Acts.

Presumably, this ideology has indeed given mental health professionals the 'necessary steadfastness and determination' through time, from being confronted by Cerletti's first patient shouting 'Not a second one! It will kill me!' to Sylvia Plath and her heroine Esther Greenwood saying 'If anyone does that to me again I'll kill myself', and on to the patient of today who simply keeps repeating 'I don't want it!', but is seen as lacking the capacity to make a decision. Once again, *Psychiatric and Mental Health Nursing* (2009), although aimed at professionals, is candid in its approach to sociology: 'mental illness is a social phenomenon rather than biologically determined.' And as for 'praise and honours', we might recall that Egas Moniz was awarded a Nobel Prize, and only a year after that, Ugo Cerletti — who was almost as widely respected — was given an honorary degree by the Sorbonne in Paris.

I believe that we should also ask ourselves whether genuinely informed consent is really possible in a psychiatric hospital situation. We have, over and over again, women and men who are demoralised and undermined by suffering and terrible sadness, entering psychiatric hospitals, which are often alarming and unpleasant and most of all *alien* environments. They are taken away from familiar surroundings and family members and they are routinely given medication in this environment, which further impairs their concentration and clarity of thought, and which in itself has the effect of making them more socially compliant and docile. Many of them may not be articulate or assertive even in the best of health. They are then urged to undergo ECT by a psychiatrist, an authority figure, who assures them that their fears are groundless and all that they have heard is rumour, and of course, a psychiatrist is a highly qualified expert. Frequently, even if they have come to hospital voluntarily, they are made to understand, either by statement or by implication, that the Mental Health Act can be used to detain them legally, in which case they can be given ECT without their consent and may have to stay in hospital for much longer.

I have spoken, over a period of more than two decades, to patients and ex-patients who were subjected to a 'good-cop-and-bad-cop' routine while under pressure to consent to ECT. The psychiatrist (frequently male) is brisk, businesslike and authoritarian, the typical bad cop, acting with a senior nurse (often female and sometimes also glamorous and feminine) who is the sweet and accepting good cop. There is, for male patients, a variation of the good cop in the form of the male nurse who plays the bluff pal: 'Come on, mate! It's no worse than going to the dentist! Tell you what, I'll buy you a pint when you're feeling better!' These adopted roles are not necessarily always calculated or cynical, they may be natural extensions of the roles played by the mental health professionals at any time.

Consent is not supposed to be obtained under duress or by undue influence. But how are these to be defined or detected or prevented? It should be painfully obvious that even extremely strong-willed people in perfect health, and with their thoughts unclouded by any medication, would find it difficult to maintain faith in their own decisions when confronted by 'experts' who may *believe* that they are doing good, especially when the environment is isolating and alien. It is in this setting that the 'mad' Catch-22 approach to mentally ill people is applied.

DOCTOR: *You are ill and suffering. You must be given ECT to make you well and stop your suffering.* PATIENT: *But I don't want ECT because it's worse than the illness. I'd rather suffer from the illness than suffer from ECT.* DOCTOR: *Ah, but you only say you don't want it because you are ill. If you were well, you would want it. When you are well, you will be grateful for it.* (Just like Hemingway, Sylvia Plath, and as many as 'one-third of individuals experiencing ECT [who] find it deeply and lastingly traumatic […] People who report benefit from ECT are in the minority'.[27] This is, perhaps, a bitter but not unjustified retort.)

It is not surprising that people with mental illnesses were seen as unfit to make a choice and as having no right to make a

---

[27] Joy Bray, 'The nurse's role in the administration of electroconvulsive therapy', in *Psychiatric and Mental Health Nursing*, edited by Phil Barker, 2nd edition, London, 2009.

Chapter One: 'History to the Defeated'

choice in the nineteenth century, when they were demonised and objectified. However, in the first decade of the twentieth century, ideas of individual liberty, autonomy, and dignity had made tremendous advances and were still advancing. The scientist and philosopher Jacob Bronowski points out that this advance had begun in the great Scientific Revolution of the seventeenth century:

> By the end of the eighteenth century, it was felt in the western world that all white men are alike; but William Wilberforce spent a lifetime in persuading his generation that black slaves and white are alike in human dignity. Science helped to create that sensibility, by widening the view of what is like and what unlike. It helped to widen it enough to make cruelty to animals a particularly detested offence in England.[28]

The understanding of what is like and what unlike kept advancing, if unevenly, extending to an acceptance of those with illnesses of the mind as simply ill, and not evil, subhuman or wilfully perverted. If moral and intellectual progress had continued fairly smoothly in this way, it would have been astonishing, almost unbelievable, to find practices such as leucotomy/lobotomy and ECT arising *and being widely accepted* as late as the 1930s. However, this progress did not continue fairly smoothly; it was shattered by the First World War, the event that led directly to the rise of fascism and Nazism and to the mental climate of the 1930s.

Taking the historical view, we can see that ideas of human liberty together with *the reality of civil liberties* were everywhere in retreat in the 1930s, and we can also see that — despite the defeat of fascism and Nazism — the world has still not entirely recovered from that retreat, even today in the early twenty-first century. In the crash of 'The Fall of Liberalism', as the historian Eric Hobsbawm calls it, in the years 1918 to 1945, 'adequately democratic political institutions' survived continuously in only five European countries — Britain, Finland, Ireland, Sweden, and

---

[28] Jacob Bronowski, *The Common Sense of Science*, London, 1951.

Switzerland.²⁹ Belief in liberty, attachment to human dignity, and a sense of the value of human life were all weakened across the whole world for decades. Accordingly, it is only too relevant to remind ourselves of the nature of the societies in which leucotomy/lobotomy and ECT were invented.

Portugal, Moniz's home country, where he carried out the first leucotomies in 1935, was the longest surviving European dictatorship, enduring from 1928 until 1974 under the rule of Antonio de Oliveira Salazar until 1968, and then under Marcello Caetano until democracy was finally established by a revolution of left-wing army officers. Portugal was a quasi-fascist state based on Catholic corporative philosophy, avoiding the leader worship and mass murder of Hitler's Germany, and yet 'without freedom or shadow of political disorder, without economic discontent or significant growth'.³⁰ It was a society that was kept in a state of artificial calm — it is tempting to say a lobotomised society. Amazingly, Moniz, a multi-talented man, was once the Portuguese foreign minister.³¹

We have seen that Cerletti's inspiration (if that is the word) for the invention of ECT came to him in a Rome slaughterhouse in 1938 in the Italy of Benito Mussolini, who was not anti-Semitic in the early years of his rule and never quite as wildly genocidal as Hitler. The loud, vulgar, and posturing Mussolini ruthlessly suppressed opponents at home and — like an unusually cowardly midget cavorting inside the vastly inflated balloon of his image — attacked defenceless small nations abroad in an effort to glorify himself. His popularity depended on theatrical bombast and upon the greed, apathy, and fear of communism of a section of the Italian population. Mussolini slaughtered fewer political enemies than Hitler, more often preferring a rubber truncheon used repeatedly on the genitals and a curiously 'medical' method of torture, namely the forcible

---

29 Eric Hobsbawm, *Age of Extremes: The Short Twentieth Century 1914–1991*, London, 1994.
30 Alan Bullock, R.B. Woodings and John Cumming, *The Fontana Biographical Companion to Modern Thought*, London, 1983.
31 Richard P. Bentall, *Madness Explained: Psychosis and Human Nature*, London, 2003.

administration of castor oil as an uncontrollable laxative for political prisoners.

Both Portugal and Italy were highly sympathetic to Hitler's Third Reich, and Mussolini became Hitler's active military ally in 1940. It is surely impossible to miss the significance of the invention of leucotomy/lobotomy and the invention of ECT only three years apart in the same dreadful decade in southern Europe and against the background of two very similar political cultures that gave rise to a similar climate of thought. (It is another of the 'ironical twists' in the history of psychiatry that Hemingway, always scathing in his contempt for Mussolini and an implacable enemy of fascism, had his literary powers destroyed by Cerletti's invention).

Once launched, of course, these methods not only fed the personal ambitions of their inventors, but also slowly acquired a commercial and economic aspect. The population of mental institutions was slowly growing with the general population in the 1930s, and with industrialisation and the expansion of the urban way of life came an increased inquisitiveness and an inquisitorial outlook on the part of many people towards their neighbours. Illnesses were now more often *diagnosed*, with the result that the sufferers were institutionalised.

Instead of the asylum doctors and nurses acting merely as jailors at worst, or caring and compassionate attendants at best, neither of which had any economic significance, there now spread the use of surgical and physical intervention, and these naturally required the production of instruments and machinery that would be endlessly elaborated. Today, we can read on the internet of an ECT machine made by Dantec Dynamics of Bristol in the UK that gives 'a synchronous, high-intensity, well-developed, and well-generalized EEG seizure pattern with a strong mid-ictal phase, pronounced postictal suppression, and a substantial tachycardia response—which is to say, an ECT-induced seizure of high expected clinical efficacy'.[32]

---

[32] See http://www.dantecdynamics.co.uk, last accessed on May 24 2010.

I began this chapter with Salvatore, the American citizen described by Dr Judith Rapoport in her book *The Boy Who Couldn't Stop Washing* (1990). Apparently, Salvatore told Dr Rapoport about the effect of his lobotomy proudly, 'now I just walk by the papers, just notice them a bit more than you might —but *I don't have to do a thing*'. This seems to me to be strangely reminiscent of the conclusion of Orwell's *Nineteen Eighty-Four* in which the tortured shell of Winston Smith finds that he loves Big Brother. If anyone thinks that I am being fanciful in introducing Orwell here, then I am in good company. Kathleen Taylor of the Department of Physiology, Anatomy and Genetics at the University of Oxford, devotes many pages to Orwell's novel in her book *Brainwashing* (2004), from which I have learned a very great deal.[33]

We must recall, yet again, the lack of theoretical justification and the lack of any test in reality, except for the reckless invasion of human bodies and personalities, which we see in the actions of Moniz and Cerletti and their successors. The words of the scientist Jacob Bronowski, spoken when he visited the museum camp at Auschwitz, sum up this kind of arrogance only too well: 'This is where people were turned into numbers […] It was done by ignorance. When people believe that they have absolute knowledge, with no test in reality, this is how they behave. This is what men do when they aspire to the knowledge of gods.'[34]

It seems to me that our society is still shaken by the reverberations of that terrible decade, the 1930s, evoked so powerfully by the poet W.H. Auden in his poem *Spain*, so full of the dread and desperate courage of the times.

> *We are left alone with our day, and the time is short, and*
> *History to the defeated*
> *May say Alas but cannot help nor pardon.*

---

[33] Kathleen Taylor, *Brainwashing: The Science of Thought Control*, Oxford, 2004.
[34] Jacob Bronowski, *The Ascent of Man*, London, 1973.

Chapter Two

The Show Takes to the Road

The huge red brick tower and chimney of Cefn Coed mental hospital, built on the outskirts of Swansea, are visible for miles in the area around the city. The poet Dylan Thomas, the only writer from Swansea to achieve international fame, describes the hospital in an early poem and letter, saying in both that it 'leers down the valley like a fool, or like a snail with […] two snail's horns'.[1] Actually, the hospital is far more imposing than Dylan Thomas suggests. The tower rises like a vast warning finger, a reminder and a symbol of authority, ever present and always to some extent permeating the consciousness and speech of the people who live in the area, so that 'in Cefn Coed' was for decades synonymous with 'mentally ill' or 'insane', and because the hospital is built on a hill, the sentence 'She'll find herself up on the hill if she goes on like that' needed no further explanation among Swansea people.

As a child, I asked about the place, and though the answer I received was sensible and humane enough, I sensed an undercurrent of dread. Since Tolkien's fantasy novel *The Lord of the Rings* attained such vast popularity in the 1970s, to be further popularised by the more recent film of the book, the hospital's appearance has inevitably been compared to the evil towers in that story (this is not a facetious invention of my own—I have met several patients and ex-patients of the hospital who have

---

[1] Paul Ferris, *Dylan Thomas*, London, 1977.

sardonically made that comparison), and any reader who has stayed with me to this point will probably grasp that this association is not merely silly or fanciful. I have, of course, dwelt upon Cefn Coed because it is the hospital of its kind that I know best, and I should add that there are many other psychiatric hospitals built in a similar style around the UK. Can we really believe that this architectural style in mental hospitals is just a coincidence (Cefn Coed was built in about 1932), or does it tell us a great deal about attitudes to mental illness and to psychiatry?

An interesting document concerning activities in Cefn Coed hospital was published in 1946. It describes the treatment by ECT of twenty-seven sufferers from *epilepsy*, twenty-five of them receiving 'regular treatment' over periods of up to seventeen months. The author of the document, Gerald Caplan, MD, BSc, DPM, formerly Deputy Medical Superintendent of the hospital, goes on to claim that for twenty-four of these people (of course, he prefers the more comforting word 'cases'), 'major fits' had been reduced, in fifteen of them to less than one third of their previous frequency. Fourteen of these people had apparently suffered from 'associated psychosis without dementia', but for all but three of them the symptoms were 'ameliorated'.

However, Dr Caplan insists that the ECT 'must be given as a form of continued replacement therapy because its effects are transient', indeed 'nine successful cases relapsed completely a few weeks after interruption of the treatment'. Nineteen cases of 'epileptic twilight state' were treated with ECT on an emergency basis and the condition was 'terminated satisfactorily' in all but one case. Nearly 1,200 ECT treatments were given (which would mean that each of these people were subjected to approximately forty-four electrically induced seizures in seventeen months or less), but Dr Caplan assures us that 'no serious or alarming complications have been experienced', and we can certainly believe that none were experienced by Dr Caplan himself.[2]

How exactly are we to understand this, even by the standards of the time? Perhaps an act of the imagination may help. Swansea was one of the towns in Britain most badly damaged by German bombing in the Second World War, and in Cefn Coed with its red brick tower rearing over the ghastly, jagged skeleton that was once the town, through the crushing grey of the winters of 1944 and 1945, undernourished and rationed and full of the greys and browns of army vehicles barrage balloons, twenty-seven pale and ill people were led to the ECT machine again and again—because they suffered from epilepsy.

How can this be understood from a medical point of view? We recall that ECT was invented as a treatment *for schizophrenia and then for depression and mania*, partly, as Professor Colin Blakemore reminds us, because of the belief that epilepsy and schizophrenia are antagonistic and incompatible. And yet here we have a description of sufferers from epilepsy being subjected to artificial, electrically induced fits. Further, this was seen as a successful treatment because it reduced the number of epileptic seizures, which do *not* erase large areas of memory of the person's life outside the period of the fit, by replacing them with ECT seizures which frequently do erase memory and arouse feelings of fear, shame, and degradation.

We must also remember that in the 1940s and early 1950s 'unmodified ECT' was given, that is *without* muscle relaxants or an anaesthetic, sometimes causing patients to suffer spinal fractures or fracture or dislocation of the long bones. Dr Caplan also insists that ECT must be given indefinitely to these twenty-seven unfortunate people and, by extension, to all epilepsy sufferers, 'as a form of continued replacement therapy because its effects are transient'—to interrupt it would cause a relapse into epileptic seizures! And these practices went on quite legally in Swansea in the last years of the war against Nazi Germany, a

---

[2] Gerald Caplan, 'Electrical convulsion therapy in the treatment of epilepsy', *Journal of Mental Science*, 92: 784–793, The Royal College of Psychiatrists, 1946.

regime that has aroused the horror of the civilised world because it exterminated or allowed obscene experiments to be performed upon the deaf, the blind, epileptics, and those with long-term mental or physical illnesses, denying them — just as it denied the Jews — any appeal, any recourse to the law, or any 'voice'.

Richard P. Bentall has been refreshingly blunt in stating unequivocally that because of this lack of a voice sufferers from mental illness 'have often been subjected to cruel and ineffective treatments [...] [T]hese have included insulin coma (which involved patients being injected with the hormone insulin, causing them to fall into a comatose state perilously close to death, whereupon they were revived and the process was repeated), and electroconvulsive therapy'.[3]

Perhaps we can exercise our imaginations once again and picture a certain scene. A large imposing building comes into view, displaying the sombre look of some kind of institution, the kind of institution that has been built to keep people in. A vehicle draws up and passes through the gates, finally stopping at the main entrance. A man with the self-important air of someone long accustomed to being treated with deference and respect gets out of the vehicle and is greeted respectfully by the head of the institution and his staff, who lead the Man of Importance to a comfortable office, while the assistants of the Man of Importance take some equipment from the vehicle and follow.

After a serious but amiable talk in the office and some refreshment, the Man of Importance goes to another room in which his assistants have set up some equipment, and along the corridor to this room members of the staff of the institution lead one of the inmates. The victim may be screaming in terror and struggling and trying to free herself, or she may be unaware of what is in store for her. She is secured to a table inside the room and the Man of Importance delivers an electric shock to her head, so that she is twitching and convulsing, but still half

---

[3] Richard P. Bentall, *Madness Explained: Psychosis and Human Nature*, London, 2003.

conscious, just like the pigs that Cerletti saw in the slaughterhouse in Rome.

Next, the Man of Importance drives a sharp instrument into her eye socket between the eyelid and the eyeball hammering it upwards into her brain with a rubber mallet, while his assistants photograph him as he does it. The victim is not dead, and the members of staff of the institution take her away. She may even meet the Man of Importance again in the future, and he may perform the procedure on her a second or even a third time.

Surely, this scene comes from a particularly cheap and unpleasant Hollywood horror film. Actually no, this is well-documented historical fact, and our Man of Importance was a real person who performed this act, not hundreds, but thousands of times.

Then perhaps we are envisaging Dr Joseph Mengele experimenting on victims in Nazi Germany, or some high-ranking torturer of the Gestapo. Sadly, this is not the case. The date of our scene is 1951, six years after the defeat of Nazi Germany, and the place is America, one of the countries that fought to defeat Hitler. The Man of Importance was Dr Walter Freeman, an American neurosurgeon of George Washington University who performed this particular form of lobotomy quite legally on thousands of psychiatric patients, and even upon recalcitrant housewives and unruly children who were not even confined to mental hospitals.

I shall refer to some of the best and most highly respected books and articles dealing with Dr Walter Freeman and lobotomy in general a little further on, as well as to an article produced for The Official Web Site of the Nobel Prize that seeks to *justify* the award of the Nobel Prize to Egas Moniz the inventor of the operation. Firstly, however, we must look a little more closely at the ways in which this operation was carried out in order to see Moniz, Walter Freeman, and other practitioners of psychosurgery in perspective.

The specific operation invented by Moniz was the prefrontal leucotomy (sometimes spelt leukotomy), involving drilling holes in the top of the skull in order to get to the brain and then severing the projections of nerve fibres that are the pathways between the frontal lobes and the rest of the brain.

Despite great advances in recent years and despite the claims of some scientists and writers—often in good faith—knowledge of the human brain is very, very partial and imperfect even today. Or rather, it would be more accurate to say that while there is now considerable knowledge of *the function of individual parts of the brain*, the way in which the brain works *as a total system* in all its varied aspects, combining thought, memory, emotion, and constantly interacting with the environment, remains almost a mystery. It does seem certain that the frontal lobes enable us to plan, to reason, to take initiatives, to possess personal autonomy and insight, to exercise self-control. The frontal lobes make us fully human and differentiate us from other animals, even the most intelligent animals, because other animals lack frontal lobes, or, as in the case of the higher apes, they are not nearly so highly developed.

After hearing the anecdote of the lobotomised chimpanzee, Moniz came up with the idea that in mentally ill people there were circuits that had stuck and jammed in the fibres that formed pathways in the brain, causing messages to be repeated in an overactive way, giving rise to morbid anxiety and agitation. There was no evidence at all to support this notion, but Moniz went ahead anyway, using an instrument called a *leucotome* that resembled a pencil with a sliding, retractable wire loop (later replaced with a steel band) to sever the nerve fibres. He found this instrument an improvement on his first technique, which involved injecting alcohol into the relevant areas of the brain in order to kill the brain tissue.[4]

The leucotomy was developed in America by Dr Walter Freeman and Dr James Watts from 1942, initially using the leucotome technique and then establishing the standard frontal

---

[4] Bengt Jansson, 'Controversial psychosurgery resulted in a Nobel Prize', http://www.nobelprize.org, The Official Web Site of the Nobel Prize, October 29 1998, last accessed on July 21 2010. Also, 'Psychosurgery: Remembering the tragedy of lobotomy', http://www.psychosurgery.org/about lobotomy/, last accessed on May 16 2010. See also, Antonio Damasio, *Descartes' Error*, below.

lobotomy that involved drilling holes in the upper forehead and cutting the brain tissue with a knife.

In his fascinating book *Descartes' Error* (1994), Antonio Damasio, Professor of Neuroscience at the University of Southern California, expresses some cautious sympathy for Moniz's experiments, while describing the Freeman and Watts frontal lobotomy as 'often a butchering affair' that was infamous 'for the questionable way in which it was prescribed and for the unnecessary mutilation it produced'.[5] This was the standard operation that was also adopted in Britain in the early 1940s, although Moniz's term leucotomy continued to be used in the UK (lobotomy is strictly speaking an American word).

However, even the standard frontal lobotomy was not enough for Dr Walter Freeman, and he soon developed the quick, convenient, and very cheap transorbital lobotomy that involved reaching the brain through the eye socket, driving a sharp instrument above the eye and through the orbit, the bone cavity within which the eye is held. He actually used an ice pick and a rubber mallet for this operation, which was not even carried out under sterile conditions.[6]

Strangely, the people subjected to the transorbital lobotomy by Walter Freeman and by others often stood the best chance of escaping the post-lobotomy changes in personality suffered by Salvatore and described in Chapter 1 above, because the neurosurgeon might fail to hit the nerve fibres altogether. These changes were noticed from the first by Moniz and then by others by the end of the 1930s, and in a symposium of 1948 the Swedish psychiatrist Gosta Rylander reported the words of a mother whose daughter had been subjected to a lobotomy: 'She is my daughter but yet a different person. She is with me in body but her soul is in some way lost. The deeper feelings, the tenderness, are gone. She is hard somehow.'[7] And only a year after Rylander's symposium, when the use of lobotomy was at

---

[5] Antonio Damasio, *Descartes' Error: Emotion, Reason and the Human Brain*, New York, 1994.
[6] Peter R. Breggin, *Toxic Psychiatry*, New York, 1991.
[7] Quoted in both Bengt Jansson and Peter R. Breggin, see fn. 4 and 6 above.

its height in both the USA and Britain, an American authority was equally unequivocal:

> These patients are not only no longer distressed by their mental conflicts but also seem to have little capacity for any emotional experiences — pleasurable or otherwise. They are described by the nurses and the doctors, over and over, as dull, apathetic, listless, without drive or initiative, flat, lethargic, placid and unconcerned, childlike, docile, needing pushing, passive, lacking in spontaneity, without aim or purpose, preoccupied and dependent.[8]

A dramatic and grotesque example of the effects on personality of damage to the brain quite similar to that inflicted by lobotomy had already come in the nineteenth century in the case of Phineas P. Gage, an intelligent, highly efficient, and courageous foreman who accidentally had a metal bar blown through his head in 1848 when supervising rock blasting. Gage survived the accident but became irresponsible, reckless, indifferent, swearing foully, unable to hold down a job, and becoming a circus freak.[9]

As we have observed, Dr Walter Freeman's transorbital lobotomy was quick, convenient, and cheap, and we should, of course, bear in mind the definition of ECT as 'a convenient and quick treatment for depression' quoted from *The Oxford Companion to the Mind* (1987) earlier. However, the extent of Walter Freeman's entrepreneurial skills — from which I took the title of the present chapter — is surprising.

In the summer of 1951, at the height of his activity in what Richard P. Bentall calls the 'manically enthusiastic' practice of lobotomy, Walter Freeman travelled across the USA and Canada in a van full of equipment (it is even said he called it his 'lobotomobile'). He moved from state to state, visiting mental hospitals, and even practising on people who were not patients.

---

[8] J.L. Hoffman, 'Clinical observations concerning schizophrenic patients treated by prefrontal leucotomy', *New England Journal of Medicine*, 241: 233–236, 1949.

[9] Antonio Damasio, *Descartes' Error: Emotion, Reason and the Human Brain*, New York, 1994.

Chapter Two: The Show Takes to the Road

Dr Freeman would subject his victims to 'unmodified' ECT, sending them into a half-conscious state of seizure, and then insert his ice pick-shaped instrument—originally an actual ice pick—under the victim's eyelid and drive it upwards through the orbit into the brain. He would sometimes demonstrate his surgical skill by driving a sharp instrument through both the patient's eye sockets at once, holding an instrument in each hand.

Walter Freeman could perform as many as twenty-five lobotomies in a day and estimated towards the end of his life that he had carried out more than 5,000 of these operations. Ironically, like many greater pioneers in history, Walter Freeman had gone through a period of profound depression as a young doctor, but this seems only to have reinforced his conviction that mentally ill people were better off with less brain function (the familiar process of objectification is always at work, it would seem, and so people are labelled according to the colour of their skin, their age, their gender, or their sexuality, and we confidently decide that they are 'better off' with less freedom and less life). [10] [11]

Walter Freeman's excesses—though not lobotomy itself—were eventually rejected, but this did not mean that the psychiatric profession cast him out, far from it. He received awards and honours and became Director of Neurology and Psychiatry at George Washington University. It is instructive to recall the insights provided by the Russian experience here, which I remarked on in the last chapter.

In 1976, the Soviet dissident Andrei Amalrik observed that those most sceptical about the political abuse of psychiatry in the Soviet Union were Western psychiatrists, because of professional etiquette and the fact that psychiatrists will always prefer to believe other psychiatrists rather than patients. Also, Solzhenitsyn had observed that those who fortify themselves with ideology (various kinds of objectification, of which psych-

---

[10] Richard P. Bentall, *Madness Explained: Psychosis and Human Nature*, London, 2003.
[11] Peter R. Breggin, *Toxic Psychiatry*, New York, 1991.

iatry is one) manage to make their actions seem good in their own eyes, so that they don't hear 'reproaches and curses but will receive praise and honours'.

The beginnings of justice were made in the case of Dr Walter Freeman when a court action for malpractice was brought against him by representatives of a woman who had suffered severe dementia due to one of his lobotomies. Dr Freeman wrote to the patient in the case, urging her to go to a hospital, because he had found that many of his lobotomised patients had committed suicide!

Dr Peter R. Breggin, who campaigned for decades to expose the nature of lobotomy, ECT, and psychiatric drugs, a professional psychiatrist not bound by the restrictions to which Andrei Amalrik referred, was to be the expert witness in the case. Walter Freeman died before the court action could be completed, and is honoured at George Washington University to this day.

Dr Freeman also recorded a taped interview that is in the archives of the American Psychiatric Association Library in which he is asked about the leucotomies performed on state hospital patients in Portugal by the man who inspired his work, Egas Moniz. 'Oh, there's plenty of Portuguese', Walter Freeman said with a laugh. Before we dismiss such callousness as an American or southern European phenomenon, we should reflect that there were obviously plenty of British as well—no less than 10,365 lobotomised patients, plus a further 762 people who were subjected to *more than one operation* between 1942 and 1954 in England and Wales.[12]

Perhaps we should pause to reflect on these figures at the risk of repetition. We should recall that 'by 1950 some 20,000 people around the world, including prisoners and children' had been lobotomised (Professor Colin Blakemore, quoted in Chapter 1 above), and that in the USA, Walter Freeman alone carried out more than 5,000 lobotomies, while in the UK in roughly the

---

[12] G.C. Tooth and M.P. Newton, *Leucotomy in England and Wales, 1942–1954*, London, 1961.

same period 11,127 people were lobotomised, including the 762 who were operated upon more than once.

What can account for such widespread use of this practice in Western democracies that were fighting or had just defeated Nazi Germany, a country that provided the terrible spectacle of what Churchill called 'the lights of perverted science'? The general reverberations of 'the fall of liberalism' to which I referred earlier must surely provide one answer, but this retreat from the commitment to human liberty and autonomy only explains how it became easier to label and objectify mentally ill people as 'unlike' the rest of us. There must be another, more immediate answer.

One writer, who defends the use of lobotomy, at least in the past, begins to supply that answer. Bengt Jansson contributed an essay entitled 'Controversial Psychosurgery Resulted in a Nobel Prize', dated October 29 1998, to The Official Web Site of the Nobel Prize. Jansson states: 'I see no reason for indignation at what was done in the 1940s, as at that time there were no other alternatives!' At first glance, this seems reasonable enough. Jansson's task is made easier—or perhaps more necessary—by the fact that in 1998 Sweden was one of the handful of countries, including the UK, that still used psychosurgery, although at the rate of only about five operations a year. Most European states had stopped using the procedure, including Finland and Norway (which gives compensation to surviving lobotomy patients). However, if we are to accept Jansson's comment we must find some result that lobotomy achieved that could not have otherwise been achieved because there was no suitable alternative.

Bengt Jansson places great emphasis on an article by V.W. Swayze.[13] This article draws attention to the sheer numbers of hospitalised mentally ill people in the USA in the 1940s: 100,000 new admissions to mental institutions and only 67,000 discharges in 1943, and nearly half of public hospital beds devoted

---

[13] V.W. Swayze, 'Frontal leukotomy and related psychosurgical procedures in the era before antipsychotics (1935–1954): a historical overview', *American Journal of Psychiatry*, 152: 505–515, 1995.

to the mentally ill in 1946. Not surprisingly, then as now, confinement in a mental hospital in itself caused illness and deterioration in personality. Jansson also takes a look at the number of people lobotomised in Britain, quoting the very figure of 11,127, and confidently reproducing the conclusions of British psychiatrists as follows. In a study conducted after the operations in order to assess their effect, it was found that out of the 9,284 patients studied 41% had 'recovered or were greatly improved', 28% were minimally improved, 25% showed no change, 2% were worse, and 4% had died.

Perhaps Jansson should have recalled Professor Blakemore's words of warning: 'the effectiveness of these operations was evaluated by the very surgeons who had invested their careers in psychosurgery: failure was not easy to accept', as well as the description of lobotomised patients already quoted above *and used in his own essay*, 'over and over, as dull, apathetic, listless, without drive or initiative, flat, lethargic, placid and unconcerned, childlike, docile, needing pushing, passive, lacking in spontaneity, without aim or purpose, preoccupied and *dependent*' (J.L. Hoffman, *New England Journal of Medicine*, 1949 — the italics are mine). Still, as there was an apparently urgent need to empty the institutions or greatly reduce the number of people in them, perhaps lobotomy was undertaken in order to achieve this. And yet, of course, this did not happen because people were so badly disabled by the operations that they remained permanently institutionalised, and only a minority were returned to their families. The typical state of post-lobotomy patients was that of the unfortunate Salvatore, a man condemned to remain in hospital.

The real reason for the popularity of lobotomy (both of the surgical kind and the more recent drug-induced equivalent) is well described by Peter R. Breggin in his book *Toxic Psychiatry* (1991), drawing upon his experience as a trained psychiatrist since 1968. Breggin quotes the lobotomist P. MacDonald Tow's revealing and ingenuous account of the state of lobotomy victims: 'the truest and most accurate way of describing the net effect on the total personality is to say that he is more simple;

and being more simple he has rather less insight into his own performance' (*Personality Changes Following Frontal Leukotomy*, 1955).

Due to these and the other effects on personality quoted above, people in mental hospitals who had been given lobotomies were dependent, easily controlled, passive, and docile, performing—as Tow puts it—'considerably better in a structured situation'. Emotionally flat and empty people make malleable and biddable psychiatric patients.

A Danish report by Heidi Hensen (1982) demonstrates that the modern forms of stereotactic psychosurgery, using electrodes to melt parts of the brain, still much recommended by psychiatrists for their precision and lesser amount of tissue damage, produce the same effect—emotional flatness, lack of initiative, and mechanical behaviour.[14] Therefore, the widespread use of this operation had little to do with relieving suffering and very little to do with reducing the population of mental hospitals. The aim of lobotomy in the USA, Britain, and every other country in which it was used (and is sometimes still used) was and continues to be the control of human beings for the convenience of others.

In the 1940s and 1950s this control was mainly exercised in the institutions, whereas today the far smaller number of people subjected to psychosurgery are more often returned—in Britain at least—to 'care in the community'. Underlying all this is the conviction that mentally ill people need to have their brain function and their personalities reduced. Jansson's claim that there is 'no reason for indignation at what was done in the 1940s' is very difficult to take seriously.

We began this chapter in the unforgiving grimness and austerity of Cefn Coed hospital, with its red brick tower rearing above bomb-shattered Swansea in the last years of the war against Hitler's Reich and the perversions it stood for. If we move on three years to another, even grimmer, institution we find the use

---

[14] Heidi Hensen *et al.*, *Stereotactic Psychosurgery*, Copenhagen, 1982.

of psychiatric practices that were equally serious and equally worth remembering.

Rampton near Nottingham was a special state institution for 'mental defectives', a category created by the Mental Deficiency Act of 1913. Together with Moss Side near Liverpool, Rampton was an institution for 'violent and dangerous' mental defectives brought from other institutions across the country or sent there by the courts. Mental defectives were further divided into three groups; 'imbeciles', 'idiots' — who would be considered today to be people with learning difficulties — and thirdly, a vague group called the 'feeble-minded'.

The individuals with learning difficulties in Rampton would often have found themselves there because they had given way to outbursts of rage due to their frustration at being unable to grasp certain basic skills, or due to open taunting by others, including teachers and their own families, which was, of course, more common and acceptable in the 1930s and 1940s. The 'feeble-minded' were people of ordinary abilities who had fallen foul of the legal system, often at an early age, and generally found it difficult to fit into society. The 'violence' of the 'feeble-minded' often consisted of nothing more dangerous to others than attempts at suicide, self-harming, or tantrums during which they broke crockery or windows. Homosexual relationships or preferences were also regarded as pathological symptoms meriting the diagnosis of feeble-minded. In 1946 there were about 60,000 'mental defectives' in institutions in England and Wales, prompting the National Council for Civil Liberties to campaign against widespread detention under the Mental Deficiency Act and against the use of those incarcerated as unpaid labour.

George W. Mackay, MB, Ch B, DPM, was Medical Superintendent of Rampton State Institution, and like Gerald Caplan, Deputy Medical Superintendent of Cefn Coed hospital, he clearly longed to share his achievements with the wider world. In 1947, George Mackay introduced the use of lobotomy/leucotomy to Rampton, writing about it in an article called 'Leucotomy in the Treatment of Psychopathic Feeble-Minded

Patients in a State Mental Deficiency Institution' a year later in 1948.[15]

The extraordinary title of this article evokes a world of attitudes, and this is intensified by the very first sentence of the piece: 'The results of leucotomy in mental hospital practice are already well known and are familiar from the Board of Control's review of 1,000 cases published in 1947.' Mackay goes on to say that in Rampton he holds some 1,200 people, he of course calls them merely 'defectives', and states that a large proportion of them are young, describing them as distinguished by 'qualities and characteristics not only of intelligence, but also by the exhibition of almost all the textbook manifestations of the psychopathic state'. The Medical Superintendent continues: 'although they *are* distinctly more intelligent, there appears to be one characteristic defect—lack of judgement and foresight [...] On the emotional side, especially among the females, there is marked instability.' And so we come once again to that dreadful instability from which women suffer—so well described by feminist historians who have written about the dealings that psychiatrists have had with women! They are not 'women' or 'young women' to Mackay, however, merely *females*, echoing the language of zoologists, or that of Nazism and apartheid.

Perhaps an act of imagination is appropriate here also, and perhaps it will not lead us too far astray. George W. Mackay, MB, Ch B, DPM, presented his article as a paper, read at a meeting of his colleagues in April 1948. A middle-aged man, well dressed and speaking with a cultured accent and a rather terse delivery—a man rather similar to Gerald Caplan, MD, BSc, DPM—would have stood in front of an audience of other men very like himself, quoting his favourite definition of the term 'Psychopathic State', published in a previous issue of *Journal of Mental Science* in an article called 'Recent Progress in Psychiatry' in 1944:

---

[15] George W. Mackay, 'Leucotomy in the treatment of psychopathic feeble-minded patients in a state mental deficiency institution', *Journal of Mental Science*, 94: 834–843, The Royal College of Psychiatrists, 1948.

> It does not imply total mental unsoundness, defect or delinquency, but yet allows for modifications of all of them — sometimes approaching the realm of defect, but yet not amounting to it — it is the name we apply to those [who have] exhibited disorders of conduct of an antisocial or asocial nature, usually of a recurrent, episodic type.

This definition, Mackay assures his listeners, describes his patients, and so he has set out to lobotomise them. Mackay's ideology — the process by which he turns those under his control into objects — makes it seem quite useful and admirable to subject them to this operation. Thus, perhaps, looking back into history and recognising parallels in the present, we can see the vast gulf that divides Mackay from his victims, the people he sees merely as *defectives, females, psychopaths, patients*. The leucotomies went on, performed upon a young man of twenty-three and a girl of fourteen among others. Mackay ends his article by stating his intention to lobotomise more patients from a larger clinical group. The category of 'mental defective' was abolished by the Mental Health Act of 1959, too late for Mackay's patients.

ECT was generally welcomed in mental hospitals in Britain from 1939 onwards, and given in 'unmodified' form, without muscle relaxants or an anaesthetic, although the frequency with which it was used varied considerably from hospital to hospital, as did the range of mental conditions for which it was prescribed.

It cannot be seriously claimed that the experience of the majority of patients who hated and dreaded the procedure varied very much. In the harsh and shabby environment of the mental hospitals of the time, smelling of urine and strong disinfectant, patients usually waited in fear outside the treatment room, which was sometimes no more than a screened off area of the ward. They would hear the sounds of their fellow patients being sent into convulsions and see them being wheeled away, still convulsing, before their own turn came. Later, they woke to numbing disorientation and confusion and memory loss.

It seems difficult to me to withhold condemnation of the attitudes and the ideology that made the use of lobotomy/leucotomy and ECT acceptable on the grounds that psychiatrists and society in general knew no better at that time. Psychiatric doctrine seems to me to be as morally reprehensible as other, strikingly similar, ideologies of the 1930s and 1940s. However, in the early 1950s, a dawn of greater awareness and enlightenment seemed to break. The age of antipsychotic drugs began.

Chapter Three

The Chemical Straitjacket

I remember a young woman sitting in the rather shabby office of the community drug advice unit I worked in, one day in the mid-1980s, with a blurred sun casting a rather brassy summer light over the city beyond the window. She was about thirty, with curly dark hair and a lovely face and figure, and although I knew something about her from a preliminary telephone conversation with her mother, I was trying to put everything else aside and focus on my own first impressions and on what she said to me.

'So how did you hear about us?' I asked the young woman —let's call her Julie—though that was not her name.

'My Mum saw an advert, and she said I should come and talk to you.'

'But *you* want to talk to me, do you? *You* would like support or advice? It's not just your Mum.' I emphasised this because it was important. I could only proceed on the basis of Julie's own wishes, not those of her mother. We gave advice and support to everyone with any kind of problem with any drug—whether prescribed, legally purchased, or illegally purchased—as long as the person concerned requested the advice.

Most of those who came to us with problems with prescribed drugs were taking benzodiazepine 'minor' tranquillisers and trying to give up these highly addictive substances and cope with the distressing withdrawal symptoms. Occasionally, however, we were contacted by people taking another class of tranquilliser called 'major' tranquillisers, usually prescribed for psychotic illnesses such as schizophrenia, not for anxiety. Julie was taking a major tranquilliser.

'Yes, OK, sure. You seem really nice.'

'Fine, Julie. And what medication are you taking?'

'Largactil', Julie said. This, I knew, was a trade name for chlorpromazine, the oldest of the major tranquillisers, one of the phenothiazine antipsychotics, and still widely used.

I was also beginning to notice things about Julie. Firstly, when I asked her a question, she would turn and make brief eye contact with me and then turn away again as she spoke, answering only the question I had asked and not elaborating on anything or volunteering anything. Secondly, her voice was flat and unemotional and her face was curiously immobile. This was, from what I had read, typical behaviour in psychotic illnesses, and it was certainly typical of every person I had met who suffered with a psychotic illness. But then, of course, every person I had met who had a psychotic illness was also taking antipsychotic medication.

'Do you remember when you were prescribed Largactil?' There was a slight hesitation before Julie answered, and two things became a little more noticeable. She was wearing a short but elegant black skirt and black boots, with one leg crossed over the other in the habitual manner of women in short skirts. Since the moment she sat down there had been a slight, rapid bouncing movement in one leg from the knee to the tip of her foot, rather like the nervous foot tapping of someone anxiously waiting, but faster and more pronounced. She also moved her head a fraction to the left about once each second. In the short pause both movements became more noticeable.

'They gave it to me when I was in hospital.' The flatness of her voice and the immobility of her face did not change.

'Do you want to tell me why you were in hospital? Don't if you don't want to.'

'I was hearing voices and getting horrible thoughts and feelings.' There was still the same cool glance, looking me in the eyes and then looking away to speak into the space in front of her.

'What about these thoughts and feelings? It's fine if you'd rather not tell me.'

'I felt as if I was being possessed by Satan and that my Mum was helping him.'

'Are you very religious, Julie?'

'No, not really.' Her face was slightly puffy, with the hint of a greasy sheen, like the face of someone who had just woken up from a night's sleep.

'So, do you still hear voices and have these thoughts and feelings now that you are taking Largactil?' I had two conflicting feelings as I asked her these questions: I am out of my depth and I can't say anything that will help her, but no, that's not quite true, if I keep my head and show uncritical support and willingness to listen, then that will be of some help, however small.

'Yes, I still hear the voices and get the same thoughts and feelings — most days, at least.' Julie's tone never changed and her face never became animated.

'Have you heard them since you've been talking to me?'

'Once or twice, Anthony, they said I shouldn't trust you or tell you anything. But I think you're OK.' This was the longest and the most personal reply she had made to me, and with it came the flicker of a smile, like the distant sweep of headlights on a winding road at night.

'Well, naturally I'll have to say that you are right and the voices are wrong.' I smiled back, and then went on. 'What, would you say, are the problems you are having with Largactil?'

'I can't feel anything — that's the problem.' Julie's answer had come swiftly and intensely for the first time.

This conversation with Julie must have made a strong impression on me, and I felt the need to write it down word for word when I got home after leaving that office, omitting her name and any details that could have identified her and locking the notebook away, not out of paranoia or any sense of my own importance, but rather out of a sense of decency and delicacy.

After the factual questions about her condition and her medication, I had tried to draw the conversation to her views and interests, mentioning my own fears, likes, and dislikes in order to encourage her. I was rather surprised that she turned up at the office to talk to me fairly often, and then attended some of our group meetings, although she said little or nothing during these encounters.

On some occasions, when talking to me face to face, she seemed livelier and more outgoing, but there were other days when she seemed worse, more withdrawn. Her mother phoned me from time to time, saying that Julie was 'a little bit better' since she had been coming to the office. However, Julie was always pessimistic when I suggested that she should discuss the effect that the chlorpromazine was having upon her with her psychiatrist, always giving the same answer: 'He says that if I stop taking the pills I'll get really ill again and be straight back in hospital.' She became friendly with two other women during the time she called at the drug advice unit, and she gradually stopped phoning me and coming to the office to talk, drifting away, either because she was growing stronger or because she was growing more despondent. I lost touch with her and never knew what happened to her in later years.

There are two things about Julie's condition that are as striking now as they were twenty-five years ago. Her psychiatrist warned her that if she stopped taking chlorpromazine she would become very ill, and yet clearly *Julie was ill even as she continued to take the drug*, judging by the fact that she still heard voices and had feelings of Satanic possession and persecution by her mother—the very symptoms that had caused her to be sent to hospital. Secondly, her physical symptoms, such as the unwanted and involuntary movements of her leg and head, were side effects of chlorpromazine and would almost certainly get worse with prolonged use of the drug. After several meetings with Julie, I thought she had taken up the habit of discreetly chewing gum, but I soon realised that this chewing motion — together with the sideways jerking of her head and the quick, bouncing twitch in her leg — was another side effect of the medication, which she had already been taking for about three years.

The *British National Formulary* (BNF), that stood on a shelf above the seat in which Julie sat during our first meeting and every subsequent meeting, is quite clear on the side effects of the antipsychotics or *neuroleptics*. (This is the prescribing guide used by GPs and other medical staff in the UK and was once rather difficult to get hold of if you were a layperson, but is now on the shelves of big book shops for anyone to buy.) I quote from the 1983 purple-covered Number 5 edition that was in the drug advice unit office at the time I knew Julie:

> CHLORPROMAZINE HYDROCHLORIDE [...] *Side-effects:* extrapyramidal symptoms (reversed by dose reduction or anticholinergic drugs) and, on prolonged administration, occasionally tardive dyskinesia; hypothermia (occasionally pyrexia), drowsiness, pallor, apathy, nightmares, insomnia, depression, and, more rarely, agitation. Anticholinergic symptoms such as dry mouth, nasal congestion, constipation, difficulty with micturition, and blurred vision; cardiovascular symptoms such as hypotension and cardiac arrhythmias; endocrine effects such as menstrual disturbances, galactorrhoea, and weight gain [...] With prolonged high dosage, corneal and lens opacities and purplish pigmentation of the skin, cornea, conjunctiva, and retina. Intramuscular injection may be painful, cause hypotension and tachycardia, and give rise to nodule formation.[1]

Before considering some definitions, so that we are absolutely clear on what the worst of these side effects really involve, and also glancing at some of the paragraphs on the preceding page in the BNF, let us notice three words that glare out of this cheerless list. The BNF advises doctors that some side effects occur with *prolonged administration* of the drug, and yet for

---

[1] *British National Formulary* (BNF), edition Number 5, British Medical Association and The Pharmaceutical Society of Great Britain, London, 1983.

decades (and still today) psychiatrists and drug companies across the world have been insisting that sufferers from schizophrenia must take the drug permanently, in order to prevent a severe relapse into their illness; that is, for life. There can hardly be any more *prolonged administration* than that! The list quoted above also informs medical professionals that these side effects occur only *occasionally*. We shall look at just what *occasionally* really means in this context a little further on.

Drugs used to treat psychotic illness, particularly schizophrenia, are variously called major tranquillisers, antipsychotics, neuroleptics, and they fall into closely related groups, most important are the phenothiazines, thioxanthenes, butyrophenones, and the drug pimozide. The drug that Julie was taking, chlorpromazine, belongs to the phenothiazine group, while another widely used antipsychotic is haloperidol, which is a butyrophenone. Some of these drugs are given in a slow release depot injection, usually fortnightly, in order to 'ensure better patient compliance', as the BNF puts it so succinctly. The same book describes what intramuscular injection of these compounds is like in the last sentence of the passage quoted above.

Today, we also have another group of drugs called atypical antipsychotics, including quetiapine and risperidone. *All* the antipsychotic drugs can cause a wide range of side effects, although some are said to be more dangerous than others, and the risk of *permanent* damage grows with the length of time the drugs are administered and with the level of the dose. *All* these drugs can cause extrapyramidal symptoms and the disease known as tardive dyskinesia. Extrapyramidal symptoms (EPS) include abnormal restlessness (akathisia), abnormal face and body movements, and symptoms resembling those of parkinsonism, an illness that causes trembling of the head and limbs, stiffness, lack of facial expression, and inability to control movements or initiate movements. Tardive dyskinesia (TD) is a disease that causes repeated, involuntary movements of the muscles controlling the face, tongue, throat, arms, and legs. The disease can develop after only a few weeks of treatment with antipsychotics on a low dosage in rare cases, but it usually occurs after some months or years of taking the drugs. Tardive dyskinesia may disappear after the drug is withdrawn, but it is more often irreversible and quite incurable.

We should also notice the warning: 'Anticholinergic symptoms such as dry mouth, nasal congestion, constipation, difficulty with micturition [that is, urinating; if we can allow that a simple word like peeing would be altogether too colloquial and plebeian for the BNF, we are still entitled to wonder why an obscure word like 'micturition' should be preferable to a familiar one like 'urinating', but perhaps the editorial committee feared that a copy might be read by patients], and blurred vision...' It is highly interesting to probe what is meant here. The part of our nervous system made up of the *cholinergic* or parasympathetic nerves controls the smooth muscles of the stomach, intestine, and bladder, making them contract. Thus, the cholinergic nerves promote digestion, salivation, urinating, and also slow the heart rate and lower blood pressure, balancing and opposing the adrenergic or sympathetic nerves that promote energetic activity.

Not only the antipsychotics or neuroleptics, but also antidepressants and lithium (a highly toxic drug used to treat manic episodes) cause *anticholinergic symptoms*, and when the drugs are withdrawn there is a *rebound* effect: previously suppressed processes return with excessive intensity. And yet the cholinergic nerves are intimately bound up with our moods and thoughts, and a rebound of their activity can cause mental disturbances. Thus, the argument that schizophrenics become ill and unbalanced when they stop taking their medication has a ready-made, circular, and self-sustaining justification.

Also, when we notice the advice that 'extrapyramidal symptoms [can be] reversed by dose reduction or *anticholinergic drugs*' (my italics) in the first lines of the passage quoted above, we seem to have arrived at some extraordinarily contorted thinking. The thinking is so contorted that we may begin to sympathise with the remark of the clinical psychologist Richard P. Bentall in *Madness Explained: Psychosis and Human Nature*

Chapter Three: The Chemical Straitjacket

(2003) that contemporary psychiatry has 'more in common with astrology than rational science'.

The general notes on antipsychotics just preceding the entry on chlorpromazine press home the message regarding the uses of these drugs and the damage they cause:

> The main use of antipsychotic drugs is in the treatment of schizophrenia where they relieve florid psychotic symptoms such as thought disorder, hallucinations, and delusions and prevent relapse [...] [L]arge doses of chlorpromazine may restore the acutely ill schizophrenic to normal activity and social behaviour where previously he was withdrawn or even mute and akinetic [...] [T]he patient who appears well on medication may suffer a disastrous relapse if treatment is withdrawn inappropriately [...] The most troublesome side-effects of antipsychotic drugs are extrapyramidal symptoms [...] These symptoms remit if the drug is withdrawn [...] Tardive dyskinesia is of particular concern because it may be irreversible on withdrawing therapy and treatment may be ineffective. It occurs fairly frequently in patients (especially the elderly) on long-term therapy and with high dosage [...] Tardive dyskinesia may also occur occasionally after short-term treatment with low dosage.

Although I have somewhat abridged this passage from the standard prescribing guide for doctors and health professionals the way in which it contradicts itself *and* the following entry on chlorpromazine will be readily seen: withdrawal of the drugs is *disastrous/necessary*; incurable tardive dyskinesia is *fairly frequent/ occasional* and so on.

In case we might think that these confusions—or this kind of treatment—were left behind in the dark days of Thatcherite Britain with its emphasis on moving patients out of hospitals into the community, its massive cuts in health spending, and its emphasis on profit, let us come right into the twenty-first century.

A comprehensive guide to drugs produced by the British Medical Association (BMA) and published in 2007 confirms that: 'antipsychotics depress the action of dopamine, they can disturb its balance with another chemical in the brain, acetylcholine. If an imbalance occurs, extrapyramidal side effects may appear [...] The most serious long-term risk of antipsychotic treatment is a disorder known as *tardive dyskinesia*, which may develop after one to five years.'[2] This book also comments on the new class of so-called 'atypical' antipsychotics such as amisulpride, clozapine, olanzapine, quetiapine, and risperidone, making it clear that with the possible exception of clozapine, these drugs may also cause tardive dyskinesia, although some of them only 'rarely'. The BNF edition of 1983 from which I have been quoting above was published after thirty years of the widespread use of antipsychotics. It remains to be seen whether the comforting word 'rarely' will still be used thirty years after the introduction of the atypical antipsychotics.

We also find that a textbook designed for use in the training of psychiatric professionals and published in 2008 deals with the subject in a much more intimate, concrete, and personal manner. There are a number of case studies at the end of the book, based on real life situations, and these studies have questions and answers attached to them. Case 9 describes a man aged fifty, living in a hostel for people with long-term mental health problems, and coming to the notice of the staff because of the odd movements he is making with his mouth and tongue. Other than this, he poses no threat, spends most of his days smoking alone, and the staff feel that 'he is quite happy in himself'.

The man spent most of the 1970s in the local psychiatric hospital and was diagnosed as a paranoid schizophrenic in 1975, but apparently he has not suffered from delusions or hallucinations in recent years. As the man is described as engaging 'very little with staff or other patients', we may wonder about the invincible optimism necessary to the conclusions that he is 'quite happy in himself' and free of delusions and hallucinations. However, the text does not invite such doubt or speculation. The man is being given injections of 150 milligrams

---

[2] Professor John A. Henry MB FRCP, editor, *New Guide to Medicines & Drugs*, 7th edition, London, 2007.

of haloperidol (an antipsychotic drug of the butyrophenone group) every four weeks—no doubt to 'ensure better patient compliance'! He is also taking 5 milligram tablets of procyclidine three times a day, which is an anticholinergic drug used to treat the parkinsonism-like symptoms caused by antipsychotics. In the text the man is given the no doubt fictional name of Mr Tomkins.

Sadly, there are thousands of people around us in the same predicament as Mr Tomkins. The book tells us that Mr Tomkins is suffering from 'residual or chronic schizophrenia', which accounts for his 'lack of motivation, social withdrawal and lack of concern for social conventions'. This teaching guide goes on to give the candid advice that the staff should be informed that the strange movements of his mouth and tongue are tardive dyskinesia caused by the haloperidol. It is fair to add that the text does suggest that the strength of the injections of haloperidol could be further reduced and that 'having injections can be unpleasant; there may be problems with the injection site as for all injections; many patients find the experience disempowering'.[3] As with another current psychiatric textbook quoted in an earlier chapter, we may feel a certain aesthetic distaste for the politically correct language employed here—the fashionable word 'disempowering' tends to obscure the fact that the experience is humiliating.

Most of us who have a little knowledge or a passing interest in the history of science or of medicine, or those of us who just proceed by common sense, would be quite justified in assuming that our understanding of the processes of the brain has steadily increased, especially our understanding of the processes of mental illness. As this understanding has expanded—we would be entitled to think—newer and better methods of *specific treatment* have been developed. Sadly, this is not the case. We have already seen that the development of lobotomy/leucotomy and ECT began with partly accidental, certainly subjective, and arguably perverse and capricious observations and inferences.

---

[3] Cornelius Katona, Claudia Cooper and Mary Robertson, *Psychiatry at a Glance*, 4th edition, Oxford/Chichester, 2008.

The history of the development of antipsychotic drugs is not very much more impressive. Worse still, when a treatment has been observed to have an effect on the mental states or personalities of people defined as mentally ill, the precise *effect* on the brain has usually been studied with eager wishful thinking. Chlorpromazine suppresses the action of dopamine in the brain by blocking dopamine receptors, and therefore it is reasoned — or rather speculated in a backwards fashion — that schizophrenia is caused by an imbalance of dopamine in parts of the brain. For rather obvious reasons, these 'treatments' are seldom tried out on those defined as sane, so that the somewhat glaring probability that their effect would be the same on anyone's brain is ignored.

The French surgeon Henri Laborit became interested in the effects of physical shock in the years following the Second World War. Shock is the result of a fall in blood pressure due to blood loss, and as well as this, injury, pain, and emotional trauma may cause a reflex widening of the blood vessels to internal organs, occurring suddenly together with a constriction of blood vessels in the skin — thus people turn 'as white as a sheet' and faint. However, Laborit was convinced that shock was more complex than this, and that it involved chemicals such as acetylcholine and histamine (the substance involved in the inflammation of body tissue). He therefore began experimenting with anticholinergic and antihistamine substances, some of them supplied to him by a large pharmaceutical company.

In 1951, while experimenting in Paris, Laborit discovered that one of these substances caused patients awaiting surgical operations to experience a lack of interest in their surroundings and emotional withdrawal. A year later, his experiments were noticed by two Parisian psychiatrists named Jean Delay and Pierre Deniker, and they were soon using Laborit's new substance on psychotic patients. This substance was shortly to be known as chlorpromazine and was used to treat schizophrenia all over the world. The large drug companies, eager as ever to make profits, began to produce substance after substance; chemically related versions of chlorpromazine, variations on the same theme.

The revolution in psychiatry was well under way. One of the central doctrines of psychiatry holds that there are a small number of psychotic illnesses, and that patients can and should be diagnosed as suffering from a *specific* psychosis and treated with a *specific* drug that is most suited to that illness. Chlorpromazine is for schizophrenia and lithium is for mania. There is a great deal of evidence that suggests that this classification is wrong. The classification is further undermined by Delay and Deniker's first 'successful' use of chlorpromazine in 1952—they gave the drug to patients who were diagnosed as suffering from mania rather than from schizophrenia.

However, we should now turn to the question of just what Delay and Deniker regarded as 'success', and I think we shall find that the answer sharply contradicts the claims made by psychiatrists over the decades since the early 1950s. In 1976, almost a quarter of a century after the first use of chlorpromazine, Dr John Pollitt, Head of the Department of Psychology, St Thomas's Hospital, made the following claim about the effectiveness of this drug in treating schizophrenia:

> In fact, even if there is some doubt about the diagnosis, it will do no harm to institute the controlling treatment [chlorpromazine]. This, we believe, induces chemical control, and stops the illness going on, helps the person to come back to interpret reality correctly, and therefore to behave appropriately, and to be able to cope independently once more [...] [W]ith every second that ticks by in which such treatment is not instituted, there is a deterioration of the personality that cannot be reclaimed. That person is being lost.[4]

Dr Pollitt's remarks should be examined in the light of history and the known facts.

---

[4] Dr John Pollitt, Head of the Department of Psychology, St Thomas's Hospital, in Tony Van Den Bergh, 'Lifelines in medicine', BBC Radio 4, reprinted in *The Listener*, September 23 1976.

A recurring feature of revolutions is the—usually brutal—candour with which the founding fathers speak of their methods and their aims, indulging in an openness that later apologists find embarrassing, and in this respect the revolution in psychiatry is no exception. Delay and Deniker wrote an account of their use of chlorpromazine in French, later published in *Congres des Medecins Alienistes et Neurologistes de France* and later translated. (In English and in French the term alienist/ *alieniste* meant someone who studied and treated mental alienation or derangement.) Pierre Deniker also published a revealing memoir in an American scholarly work in 1970.[5]

Reading the account written by these pioneers gives a startling sense of recognition to those of us who have known patients taking antipsychotics. They say of these first patients to be given chlorpromazine *in doses that were small by later standards* that they remained: 'silent most of the time [...] [I]f questioned [they] answer slowly and deliberately in a monotonous and indifferent voice; [they] express themselves in a few words and become silent.'

As we have seen, the use of chlorpromazine quickly spread across the world, and a further report was written by a Canadian called Heinz Lehmann and published in *Archives of Neurology and Psychiatry* in 1954. Lehmann observed that: 'the patients under treatment display a lack of spontaneous interest in the environment.' And contrary to the assertions that were put about in later decades and still today, Lehmann stated that chlorpromazine had no 'direct influence [...] on delusional symptoms or hallucinatory phenomena'.

The use of this drug and other antipsychotics in Britain is usually dated from 1954, and in that year D. Anton-Stephens published a report in the *Journal of Mental Science* quoting the same 'indifference' and apathy as the consistent effect produced by these substances. This was echoed by the Americans Arthur Noyes and L. Kolb in the 1958 edition of their book *Modern Clinical Psychiatry*: indifference to the patient's inner and outer

---

[5] F. Ayd Jr. and B. Blackwell, editors, *Discoveries in Biological Psychiatry*, Philadelphia, 1970.

world was the response that psychiatrists wished to produce when they administered chlorpromazine and the compounds related to it. Later, extravagant and would-be humane descriptions of the therapeutic value of the antipsychotic drugs became the norm, until the whistle was blown—so to speak—by a neuroanatomist named Peter Sterling of the University of Pennsylvania. Writing in the *New Republic* of March 3 1979, Sterling stated: 'the influence of chlorpromazine resembles nothing so much as the effects of frontal lobotomy.'

It is, of course, the psychiatrist Peter R. Breggin who has done most to expose the use of antipsychotic or neuroleptic drugs as 'chemical lobotomy', particularly in his admirably readable and very moving book, *Toxic Psychiatry* (1991). Clearly, these chemicals became immensely popular for a number of reasons, including the drive for profits on the part of the drug companies, and it is not difficult to see that it is easier to market 'miracle drugs' successfully than it is to market lobotomies or even ECT machines.

The use of antipsychotics, like the use of lobotomy, made people passive, biddable, and easier to control. Undoubtedly, there was also the genuine belief on the part of some psychiatrists and nurses that they were doing good and relieving suffering. The whole process was made easier by the ever present objectification of others—in this case people with mental illnesses—of which human beings are so obviously capable. There is one other dreadful possibility, an awful historical parallel, which I will tentatively suggest.

The widespread and frequent use of lobotomy and of ECT, and particularly the use of the even more brutal, 'unmodified' ECT of the 1940s and 1950s, requires a large number of staff with the necessary firmness, dedication, and belief in what they are doing. But the results of lobotomy and ECT are only too visible and obvious to those who carry out such procedures, particularly when they are inflicted upon patients against their will. It surely becomes difficult to go on deceiving yourself. And it is here that there arises the possibility of a ghastly parallel.

The development of the gas chambers was welcomed by leading Nazis *not only* because it provided a more efficient method of exterminating the Jews, but *also* because it made things easier for the exterminators. The Nazi leaders were concerned that even trained SS men would be unable to cope with the task of the mass shooting of men, women and children, day after day.

Did the introduction of the antipsychotics fulfil some kind of comparable function? Is it not easier to justify giving medication than to justify performing brain operations or producing repeated convulsions by electricity? The psychiatrists Peter R. Breggin and Thomas Szasz had little doubt that this is the case. Breggin remarks that the antipsychotic drugs 'salved the consciences of psychiatrists and made them feel more like legitimate doctors'. Szasz ironically comments: 'Restraint by chemical means does not make us guilty; herein lies the danger to the patient.'[6] These writers did not explicitly draw the parallel between the psychological usefulness of lethal gas to the architects of the Holocaust and the psychological usefulness of antipsychotic drugs to the psychiatric profession. I must leave it to the individual reader to decide whether or not this parallel is unduly fanciful or grotesque.

We have already had cause to consider the Soviet experience of psychiatry in an earlier chapter. In the 1970s, the Soviet authorities arrested the scientist Leonid Plyushch because, like many Russian intellectuals, he had developed political views that were critical of the Soviet system. Also, like other dissidents at that time, Plyushch was confined in a psychiatric hospital and given forcible treatment with drugs. He was later released and able to come to the West, where he spoke to the media, recalling with horror the effect upon him of the drugs he had been given: 'I deteriorated intellectually, morally and emotionally from day to day. My interest in political problems quickly disappeared, then my interest in scientific problems, and then my interest in

---

[6] Thomas Szasz, 'Some observations on the use of tranquilizing drugs', *Archives of Neurology and Psychiatry*, 77: 86–92, 1957.

my wife and children.' On February 14 1976, *The New York Times* quoted some of the more specific information given by Plyushch to the Western media regarding his experiences: 'I was prescribed haloperidol in *small doses*' (my italics).

As I write this, I have side by side before me the teaching textbook that we looked at above, *Psychiatry at a Glance* (2008), and a review by A.V. Campbell of a book called *The Case of Leonid Plyushch*—a review that was rather ironically published in the *Journal of Medical Ethics*. Campbell begins by saying that the success of the film *One Flew Over the Cuckoo's Nest* 'seems to be an indicator of a growing public awareness of the ambiguity of the concept of mental illness and of the potentially exploitative uses of psychiatric treatment'. Further on, just like *The New York Times*, Campbell repeats Plyushch's testimony that 'haloperidol, insulin and other drugs were administered' to him.[7]

However, if we recall the unfortunate Case 9 in the psychiatric textbook, 'Mr Tomkins', aged fifty, we will see that he was also being given that very same drug, haloperidol (closely related to chlorpromazine). Mr Tomkins' 'lack of motivation, social withdrawal and lack of concern for social conventions' are of course ascribed to his 'residual or chronic schizophrenia' in our textbook, but not to the 150 milligrams of haloperidol with which he is being injected every four weeks. Plyushch, however, specifically links his loss of interest in politics, in his scientific work, and even in his wife and children to being forcibly drugged with haloperidol. But Leonid Plyushch was a renowned mathematician and scientist and a very brave man, as well as a victim of the enemies of the West, whereas Mr Tomkins and the thousands like him do not give international press conferences or attract the notice of *The New York Times*.

It was much easier to react with indignation and horror to the effects of drugs like haloperidol when they were used in the Soviet Union in the 1970s, just as it is much easier in the first decade of the twenty-first century to condemn the brutality of

---

[7] A.V. Campbell, 'The case of Leonid Plyushch', review, *Journal of Medical Ethics*, 2 (4): 211, December 1976.

Russia in pursuing its strategic interests than to recognise that the West is acting with similar ruthlessness.

The psychiatric teaching guide also informs us that Mr Tomkins was an in-patient in a psychiatric hospital for most of the 1970s and was diagnosed with paranoid schizophrenia in 1975 — the very time that Plyushch was undergoing his ordeal.

The antipsychotic or neuroleptic drugs make people perform 'better in a structured situation', as was once said about lobotomy, and in the case of Russian dissidents, that 'structured situation' was Soviet society itself. The benefits of the surgical or chemical lobotomy to psychiatrists, doctors, nurses, social workers, warders, teachers, and family members are not difficult to see.

There is fascinating evidence that demonstrates that far from *specifically* acting upon the symptoms of schizophrenia or other psychotic illnesses, the so-called antipsychotics are no more beneficial than other simple sedatives. According to the *American Journal of Psychiatry* (October 1989), in which Paul Keck and Ross Baldessarini reviewed five studies that compared neuroleptics to other drugs or with simple placebos, the 'antipsychotic' drugs were no more effective than diazepam (Valium) or opium — the same overall improvement over four weeks of treatment was observed in the case of these substances.

I personally remember a young man who was being given fortnightly injections of an antipsychotic called flupentixol, which he disliked and regarded as of no help to him. He did, however, find a good deal of relief in taking diazepam, regarded as only useful for moderate anxiety and depression. This was in the 1990s, when benzodiazepines such as diazepam had been recognised as highly addictive, and for this reason his GP would only prescribe very small amounts of the drug — yet antipsychotics with their dangerous and incurable side effects are promoted as drugs to be taken for life in order to prevent 'a disastrous relapse'! It is also objected that diazepam is 'nonspecific', yet the neuroleptics are no more specific. Peter R. Breggin puts it with his usual forthrightness:

> The neuroleptic drugs are chemical lobotomizing agents with no specific therapeutic effect on any symptoms or problems [they] blunt and subdue the individual [...] [T]hey also physically paralyze the body, rendering the individual less able to react or move [...] [T]hey produce a chemical lobotomy and a chemical straitjacket.

If the much publicised therapeutic effect of halting the process of schizophrenia that has been claimed for the antipsychotic drugs is illusory and deceitful, then how widespread are the side effects caused by these drugs? In 1980, more than a quarter of a century after the introduction of neuroleptics across the world, the American Psychiatric Association's official task force for investigating tardive dyskinesia (TD) published its report. The figures are, frankly, shocking. Some ten to twenty per cent of patients receiving antipsychotic medication for a period of six months to two years would develop the disease, and in older people and for those receiving the drugs for longer periods the number of victims of TD rises to forty per cent in hospitals, and increases yet again among elderly women patients (the very section of the community most subjected to ECT against their will).

Breggin quotes the Canadian Guy Chouinard in *Clinical Psychiatry News* (June 1990): 'drug exposure of fifteen years and more would lead to almost certain risk for tardive dyskinesia.' Breggin's book, *Toxic Psychiatry* (1991), also recounts the — entirely predictable — story of denial, rejection, and manipulation of information on the part of psychiatrists, partly motivated in the USA (which has a more extensive anti-establishment litigation tradition than Britain) by fear of legal cases for malpractice.

The true figures for the incidence of tardive dyskinesia are almost certainly higher than those given in earlier official studies because of a number of factors, including the increasing use of depot injections of antipsychotic drugs. (We should recall that *supervised community treatment orders* were introduced in the 2007 Mental Health Act in Britain, and those subject to those orders who refuse treatment can be taken to hospital and treated against their will.) Considerable numbers of people taking antipsychotic drugs in the form of pills, whether in hospitals or in the community, may have avoided taking them temporarily or permanently, but this is not the case with injected preparations.

Other factors that have distorted earlier findings include the very brief time spent examining patients and the fact that people are monitored only for the duration of a study, even if this extends over months or two or three years—patients who are free of tardive dyskinesia while the study is being conducted may well develop it later. The figures march on, and based on the number of Americans prescribed antipsychotics since the 1950s, a figure of a million tardive dyskinesia sufferers in the USA in the 1990s seems reasonable.

According to Breggin and the British psychologist David Hill, the drug company Roche estimated that there were 150 million people taking antipsychotic drugs worldwide in 1980. This figure was used by Hill to estimate that across the world 'some 38.5 million people are currently suffering from tardive dyskinesia'.[8] (These drugs are not, of course, given only to those labelled schizophrenics, but also to hyperactive children, elderly people in nursing homes, those with learning difficulties, and prisoners.) The figure may be only half that much—which is highly unlikely—or it may be twice as much, but numbers of this magnitude constitute an artificially created epidemic of historic, perhaps unique, proportions.

I have already remarked upon the inverted speculative reasoning that has arisen from the observed effect of antipsychotics: the drugs subdue and blunt the reactions of those diagnosed as schizophrenic by suppressing the action of dopamine in the brain and *therefore* schizophrenia must be *caused* by an imbalance of dopamine. This is about as sensible as the notion that because people are notoriously more likely to have casual sex after several drinks on a Saturday night, sexual inhibitions or

---

[8] David Hill, 'Opinion: The problem with major tranquillisers', *Openmind*, No. 13, February/March 1985.

scruples must be *created and caused* by an insufficiency of alcohol in our brains. This faulty reasoning is further reinforced by the fact that the suppression of brain processes, anticholinergic or dopamine blocking, causes a compensatory *rebound* effect—so that yes, schizophrenics who have been given neuroleptics have high levels of dopamine activity.

There is also the fact that excitement and intense emotion immediately influence the levels of chemicals and the kind of electrical waves in the brain. The biological basis of 'madness' has continued to be a persistent and elusive goal for psychiatrists despite these painfully obvious objections.

It is worth quoting Richard P. Bentall once again for his comments on this quest for the biology of mental illness that has been met by 'a dramatic suspension of the critical faculties of both researchers and bystanders […] [D]iscoveries are announced triumphantly, [researchers have an] unreflective hunger for the rewards and plaudits that go with genuine scientific progress […] as if they are Mesmerized by the scent of the Nobel Prize' (*Madness Explained: Psychosis and Human Nature*, 2003). How accurate a description this is of Egas Moniz and Ugo Cerletti, the originators of lobotomy and ECT, leaving a legacy of misery and mutilation stretching over decades!

Schizophrenia, Breggin points out, 'has been called madness […] [I]ts often flamboyant psychospirituality combine[s] with its typically overwhelming feelings of fragmented identity, humiliation, and helplessness […] Instead of offering human understanding […] psychiatry has fabricated biological and genetic explanations […] to justify a massive drug assault that has taken a profound toll in terms of damaged brains and shattered lives'. I suggest that this account of schizophrenia, consistent with the facts about the real nature of treatment by antipsychotic drugs, demonstrates that the remarks of Dr John Pollitt of St Thomas's Hospital in 1976—quoted above and echoed repeatedly right up to the present—are a naïve, vulgar, and self-serving flight from reality.

Since the 1950s, when the neuroleptic drugs were introduced, the number of drugs prescribed for mental illness has gone on increasing: tricyclic antidepressants, monoamine oxidase inhibitor antidepressants, the highly toxic substance lithium for mania, and the newer selective serotonin re-uptake inhibitor antidepressants such as fluoxetine (Prozac) and escitalopram (Cipralex). All of them have serious side effects — in some cases the severity of these cannot yet be fully assessed — and all of them are used as a substitute for 'offering human understanding'.

These substances are believed to act on the *specific biochemistry* of mental states in the same way as the neuroleptics are believed to halt the process of schizophrenia, and yet again effect (usually not a very good effect) is confused with some hypothetical cause. The manufacturers shrewdly tell us that antidepressants can take a month or several months to have their effect, which quietly avoids mentioning the fact that between a quarter and a half of people who are severely depressed will recover without treatment within a few months. Depressed people who recognise that they have a problem begin to make some kind of change in their lives, talk to others and reach out to others, are even more likely to recover spontaneously. Meanwhile, the 'miracle drugs' are given the credit, the drug companies rake in the profits, and the psychiatric profession increases in power and prestige.

Chapter Four

Suitable Cases for Study: Psychiatry in Literature and Film

George Orwell remarked, in an essay written in 1944, 'during the past decade and more, things have been happening to middle-class people [in continental Europe] which in England do not even happen to the working class'. He was thinking of the collapse of liberal democracy and the spread of fascism in one European country after another, and it was to this that he attributed the superiority of European political literature.[1]

Something of the same is true of the literature of mental illness and mental hospitals. Not only had the subject matter of literature broadened so that this issue could be written about in the twentieth century (in Russia, Anton Chekhov had already dealt with it in *Ward 6* in 1892), but also — partly because ECT and neuroleptic drugs made psychiatrists 'feel more like legitimate doctors' as Peter R. Breggin put it — asylums were now seen as humane hospitals. Thus, middle-class intellectuals and writers came into contact with *pockets or islands* within Western society in which people who had committed no crime were subjected to a profound loss of liberty. This contact often took the form of writers finding themselves the victims of that loss of

---

[1] George Orwell, 'Arthur Koestler', *The Collected Essays, Journalism and Letters*, Volume 3, London, 1968.

freedom, and sometimes they became familiar with it because they were temporarily employed by the system.

The short selection of books and films in this chapter is inevitably incomplete and arbitrary, and it includes works of varying quality, but hopefully, for anyone interested in the subject of my own book, some of the most interesting examples will be found here.

One Flew Over the Cuckoo's Nest by Ken Kesey (1962)

Ken Kesey's novel is the one book about mental hospitals and mental illness that almost everyone — even those who have never taken any interest in the subject — has heard of, if not read. Its popularity was given an immense boost by the 1975 film of the same name, directed by Milos Forman and starring Jack Nicholson. In fact, Jack Nicholson has become so inextricably associated with McMurphy, the central character of both book and film, that British paperback editions carrying Nicholson's photograph in the role are still being sold today.

The novel is set in 1960, the year in which Kesey, then a student aged twenty-four, had volunteered to take part in government funded experiments with mood changing drugs at Menlo Park Hospital. He later worked for a time as a nurse's aide in the same mental hospital, developing a sympathy and a sense of affinity with the patients. The book and film have entered the popular consciousness, dealing a permanent blow against social control and conformity imposed by psychiatric means, just as Orwell's novel *Nineteen Eighty-Four* dealt a permanent blow against the dictatorship of what we now call 'the surveillance society', making it more difficult for that society to establish itself and flourish.

The main action of the book takes place in a ward of a mental hospital, run with merciless efficiency by Miss Ratched, the Big Nurse, whose name suggests 'ratchet' — she is frequently described as metallic, machine-like. Names are important in the allusive, modernist text of the novel, sometimes deliberately parodying earnest psychological techniques such as verbal association and the compulsive habit of verbal association found in mental illness. An immature younger patient, whose development is undermined by both Miss Ratched and his own mother, is called Billy Bibbit (Bunny Rabbit, and a 'bib' as worn by a baby), while the sexually inadequate Harding, the most intellectual and educated of the patients, is ironically quite lacking in 'hardness', either in the sense of physical toughness or sexual potency.

The main features of this ghastly setting—what one advocate of lobotomy called 'a structured situation'—are humiliation and crushing tedium. The ward is suddenly invaded by Randle Patrick McMurphy (rpm, revolutions per minute, randy, mirth, mercy), a brawling, gambling, wandering man who has feigned mental illness in order to get himself transferred from the hard labour regime of the local prison. He feels delighted with the success of the trick he has played as he arrives in the ward. The narrator of the story reflects that McMurphy is 'hard', not in the way of the narrator's own father (a Native American chief) who was 'hard and shiny as a gunstock', but 'hard in a different kind of way from Papa, kind of the way a baseball is hard under the scuffed leather'. The 'baseball' is shortly to collide with metallic, machine-like Miss Ratched.

The narrator of *One Flew Over the Cuckoo's Nest* is Chief Bromden, a man who is six feet and eight inches tall, whose father was a Native American from Columbia, and whose mother was a white Christian. The Chief is suffering from some kind of mental illness, presumably triggered by his experiences as a frontline soldier in the Second World War, and he has been a patient in the hospital for many years, pretending to be deaf and mute—'being cagey'—in order to avoid attention. He has good reason to avoid the attention of the hospital staff, having been given more than two hundred ECT treatments, and is indeed ignored as long as he gets on with sweeping the ward, living up to his nickname, Chief Broom. (In case the figure of two hundred unmodified ECT treatments seems an unlikely one, I must point out that we shall encounter that figure again a little further on in a non-fiction account of impeccable integrity.)

Despite his mental problems—or what may be simply the damage done by ECT—Chief Bromden has an intuitive and visionary grasp of reality that no other character in the book can equal, and in fact this kind of clarity of perception is often exhibited by those labelled mentally ill in real life. Only the Chief fully grasps that the real problem is not Miss Ratched, but rather society itself, which he calls the Combine, demanding conformity and seeking control over us, so that the Big Nurse 'is just a high-ranking official'.

Chief Bromden is the only character who notices the real complexity of McMurphy's personality that exists alongside his laughing, swaggering toughness: he paints a wonderful picture spontaneously during Occupational Therapy; he writes letters in beautiful, flowing handwriting 'to somebody'; he is 'upset and worried' when he receives a letter in reply; at moments when he thinks he is unobserved, McMurphy's face is 'dreadfully tired and strained and *frantic*', and later 'thin and scared'.

While Harding speaks for Ken Kesey, the university educated intellectual, and provides us with a link to the common sense, rational world, Chief Bromden expresses the intuitive wisdom of the artist and the compassion of the individual who has survived hideous suffering. The Chief is also a mutilated warrior prince in captivity—as in the Samson legend with which I began this book—as well as one of the victims of American society simply because of his race. His name, Bromden, suggests 'brooding' and 'brewing' and 'promise', and it also suggests 'bomb'—he is haunted by air raids because of his wartime experiences—and he is indeed the unexploded bomb of self-assertion and rebellion in the story.

The demeaning nickname Chief Broom reminds us of the mundane and humble implement that he constantly uses. However, in folklore and legend the humble broom can become an instrument of magical power. The Chief has been pointlessly and ineffectually sweeping and cleaning for years, and yet he only begins to sweep away the moral 'poisons' and 'mess' that he so clearly perceives when he has been regenerated by McMurphy's influence.

Chapter Four: Suitable Cases for Study

McMurphy is second only to the Chief in intuitive understanding, but McMurphy's intuition is the cunning of the active survivor, not the passive survivor, deriving from the split-second reactions he has needed as a gambler, a street fighter, and a con man. He only comes to share most of Chief Bromden's insights at the very end of the novel, after much suffering and on the brink of his own destruction.

After his arrival in the ward, McMurphy's euphoria over leaving hard labour behind quickly turns to bewilderment at the ritual humiliation of the Group Therapy Meeting in which one patient—any patient, but in this instance Harding—is subjected to questioning and insinuations by the others, carefully orchestrated by Miss Ratched. McMurphy cannot understand why grown men participate in such a spectacle. He is quickly advised that any *overt* aggression, hostility, or dissent can lead to confinement on the Disturbed Ward, forcible ECT, or even a lobotomy. At this point, McMurphy bets his fellow patients that he can break through Miss Ratched's icy control, make her angry, make her look silly, and undermine her authority. He spectacularly succeeds a week later.

Kesey's novel overwhelmingly depicts oppression in the mental institution as *the oppression of men by women*, and this is not in itself incredible or untrue. Sexuality and sexual identity have frequently been seen as one of the most dangerous attributes of mentally ill people, requiring suppression or removal. There were—and are—tyrannous women who see part of their function within the psychiatric system as carrying out just this kind of suppression and removal, no doubt providing an outlet for their own conflicts and grievances. Also, men have notoriously found opportunities within the psychiatric system to satisfy their appetites for exercising control over women.

However, there is not a single phrase in *One Flew Over the Cuckoo's Nest* that even acknowledges the existence of women mental patients, let alone acknowledging their sufferings. This is a serious lack of balance and perspective in the novel, despite the appearance of humane and decent female characters such as the Japanese nurse on the Disturbed Ward, the Afro-American women factory workers of Chief Bromden's reminiscences, and—most decent and humane of all—the two prostitutes who are friends of McMurphy.

The issue of race, parallel with the gender issue, is treated with considerably more depth and subtlety, although McMurphy's and Chief Bromden's use of racist language can understandably mislead readers on this point. As we have seen, the novel's narrator is a Native American, a victim of the American system, and yet Miss Ratched's three Afro-American aides are the most unrelentingly evil characters in the story. However, these aides are also victims, and it is explicitly stated that one of them has witnessed his parents being raped and tortured when he was still a child. The quality that Big Nurse appreciates in these men is the very hatred that persecution has aroused in them, so that she can utilize it and channel it. The parallels with all political systems and institutions that require trusted servants to exercise unhesitating control over other human beings are almost too obvious. In sharp contrast, the Afro-American aide Mr Turkle, who works the long night shift on the ward, is a kindly and decent man, although full of ordinary human weaknesses. Finally, of course, despite all her power, Miss Ratched is also a dreary servant of the system with which she has identified herself.

The pivotal moment of the novel comes soon after McMurphy's outstanding success in reducing Miss Ratched to ineffectual, screaming rage. He has naïvely expected to serve out his original short prison sentence in the mental hospital, but he is now informed that he has been committed and must remain there for an indefinite time until the hospital authorities (including and especially Miss Ratched) decide to release him.

However, the truly shocking revelation is that almost all of his fellow patients are there on a voluntary basis—they can leave any time they wish. *'Why?* [...] why do you stand for it?' McMurphy rages at them. The answer is that they are simply too weak and inadequate to face life outside the hospital. And yet the hospital is only a concentrated microcosm of society and the voluntary patients are only exaggerated versions of ordinary citizens—as Chief Bromden sees quite clearly—and so the message of the book is one that passes judgement on all of us: why do we stand for it? Far from turning his back on the other patients, McMurphy decides to resume his struggle with the Big Nurse at this moment, so that what has begun as the dangerous game of an adventurer, and the wager of a compulsive gambler turns into a deadly duel with authority.

Miss Ratched is dehumanised and tyrannous, but she is not stupid. Together with Chief Bromden, McMurphy, and Harding, she is the fourth character in the novel capable of piercing insight, and because of this she does not underestimate McMurphy, regarding him instead as a formidable threat. McMurphy has also been warned of the dangers of defying the system. Harding describes ECT:

> [Y]ou are jointly administered therapy and a punishment for your hostile go-to-hell behaviour, on top of being put out of everyone's way for six hours to three days, depending on the individual. Even when you do regain consciousness you are in a state of disorientation for days. You are unable to think coherently. You can't recall things [...] Absolutely painless. The thing is, no one ever wants another one. You... change. You forget things.

As both McMurphy and the Big Nurse choose, so to speak, to *ratchet up* the conflict, McMurphy's awareness of impending disaster increases, although the signs of this are seen only by Chief Bromden. In the film version McMurphy finally resorts to violence in a moment of accidental exasperation, but in the book he quite explicitly uses violence to protect one of the other patients from torment and humiliation, realising the consequences of his actions with 'helpless, cornered despair'.

Miss Ratched is shrewd enough to bargain with McMurphy at this point, asking him to apologise for his actions—thus destroying his credibility with the other patients and restoring her authority—as an alternative to ECT. McMurphy refuses and is subjected to repeated treatments, pretending by a huge effort of will that they do not affect him. Chief Bromden is the only one who joins in McMurphy's physical fight with Ratched's aides in defence of a fellow patient, and because he is once again subjected to ECT he also understands the extent of McMurphy's suffering. The Chief tells us: 'The thing he was fighting, you couldn't whip it for good. All you could do was keep on whipping it, till you couldn't come out any more and somebody else had to take your place.'

The film concentrates McMurphy's possible escape from the ward (after a riotous and anarchic night on which he has smuggled the two prostitutes Candy and Sandy armed with a large amount of liquor into the hospital) into a moment by a window unlocked with stolen keys. He is shown as fully prepared to leave in the film, only returning to try to strangle Miss Ratched because she has gratuitously goaded Billy Bibbit into cutting his own throat.

There is no such clear turning point in the novel, which shows McMurphy being presented with even more ample opportunities for escape. He claims to be too drunk to leave, but is clearly unwilling to do so because he has resigned himself to continuing the struggle and to his own destruction.

After being overpowered in his attempt to strangle the Big Nurse, McMurphy is taken away and given a lobotomy, returning to the ward as a vegetating shell of his former self. Chief Bromden smothers what is left of McMurphy as the lobotomised victim sleeps, and then makes his own escape from the hospital that has confined him for more than fifteen years.

The differences between the novel and the film highlight one of the most exciting themes in academic film studies, namely defining *what constitutes* a film adaptation. The critic Geoffrey Wagner, in a contemporary approach to this effort at definition, names three main kinds of adaptation. A direct transposition of a literary work onto the screen (such as the rendition of a novel in cinematic form that is intended to be an illustration of the original text, even containing an opening shot of the title page) is distinguished from a commentary, which is a cinematic story with many points of similarity and many points of divergence from a literary work. These are further distinguished from a film that is only an analogy, having a very tenuous connection to a literary text, sometimes little more than bearing the same title or a similar title.[2]

The film based on Ken Kesey's novel must finally be seen as a commentary, and yet film and book have fused in the popular imagination, creating a permanent and widespread wariness of psychiatric practice. The film is superior to the book, for example, in its depiction of ECT because of the greater realism and exactness with which this is presented on the screen.

Does the novel have any continuing relevance for us today, whatever its virtues as a piece of literature or a portrait of America in 1960? We may answer this question with a shrug: well, things were so very different in those days. I believe that answer to be mistaken. As Richard P. Bentall points out in *Madness Explained: Psychosis and Human Nature* (2003), our own British psychiatric wards in the twenty-first century present a cheerless spectacle: 'the overwhelming impression is one of inactivity and loneliness [...] [P]atients sit in the ward lounge, silently smoking cigarettes, their faces glued to daytime television shows [...] [N]urses [...] spend most of their time in the nursing office.' This description is eerily familiar to anyone who has read *One Flew Over the Cuckoo's Nest*. Cruelty may flourish through the apathy, unimaginative routine, demoralization, and wish for convenient solutions on the part of medical staff in such an environment, just as it flourished in a more deliberate and calculated way in the world of Miss Ratched.

Circumstances and conditions change, but the essence of oppression sometimes persists. In Joseph Conrad's novel *The Secret Agent*, published in 1907 and set in the London of 1886, a terrorist known as the Professor walks the streets with explosives strapped to his body, ready to blow himself up and those around him, dreaming of the perfect detonator, while the representative of a foreign government and a secret agent indulge in the moral filthiness of arranging a terrorist incident for political gain. We would be foolish, for the most obvious reasons, if we were to dismiss this novel as a gripping tale of the

---

[2] Geoffrey Wagner, *The Novel and the Cinema*, New Jersey, 1975.

past without relevance to the world of today. It would be equally naïve, I believe, to think of *One Flew Over the Cuckoo's Nest* as merely a description of horrors we have left behind us.

The Bell Jar
by Sylvia Plath (1963)

Kesey's McMurphy, and also Harding, draw an explicit connection between ECT and execution in the electric chair, a connection that was made equally explicit by the New Zealand novelist Janet Frame, whose writing we shall look at a little further on. Sylvia Plath (1932–1963) begins her novel *The Bell Jar*: 'It was a queer, sultry summer, the summer they electrocuted the Rosenbergs, and I didn't know what I was doing in New York.' (Ethel and Julius Rosenberg were executed at Sing Sing Prison on June 19 1953 as Soviet spies, although the prosecution case was based on testimony of doubtful reliability, and even though the alleged spying had taken place during the Second World War when the Soviet Union was an ally of the United States.)

Thus Plath's narrator, Esther Greenwood, who cannot stop thinking about the Rosenbergs, sets the tone for the story that follows: authoritarian and institutional cruelty, Cold War America, and the society of the 1950s with its stifling restrictions on female fulfilment.

Sylvia Plath was to become a heroine to the women's movement because feminists saw her as a victim of patriarchy, but it should be noticed that Sylvia's/Esther's mother, Mrs Plath/Greenwood, is one of the main causes of her problems, and also connives with the psychiatric system. Also, the main positive female character in *The Bell Jar*, the psychiatrist and surrogate mother Dr Nolan—Dr Ruth Beuscher in real life—is far from unambiguously benign.

Dr Beuscher was to remain Plath's guide, adviser, and therapist for the rest of her life, although she could not or would not respond to Plath's desperate pleas and come to London in the months before Plath killed herself in that city on February 10 1963. Thus Beuscher seems to have repeated the pattern of the mother who creates dependence and then abandons her child at a crucial moment, which is a recurrent theme in psychiatric literature.

Mrs Greenwood, Esther's mother in *The Bell Jar*, is as suffocatingly undermining as Billy Bibbit's mother in *One Flew Over the Cuckoo's Nest*, and it is, of course, instructive to look at *The Bell Jar* alongside Kesey's novel, which—as we have seen—ignores the existence of women mental patients and their sufferings. Sylvia Plath's book often has as much stylistic richness as *One Flew Over the Cuckoo's Nest*, though little of its pace, drama, and brutality.

The novel seems to follow the events of Sylvia Plath's own life so closely that some critics have doubted whether it should be called a novel at all, and it was presumably because of the autobiographical aspect that she published it under the pseudonym Victoria Lucas when it appeared in Britain in 1963. I do not think that in literary terms the distinction between autobiographical novel and autobiography means very much, if only because writers have always written one genre and called it the other.

It is, of course, the book's fidelity to actual events that gives it even greater value in the literature of mental illness and psychiatry. Esther Greenwood is in New York because—like Sylvia Plath—she has won a competition for young writers, one of the prizes for which is the chance to work on a top magazine in the city, with all expenses paid. The experience turns sour, and Esther's emotions become increasingly fragile, even before the socialising, agonizing over losing her virginity, and the dating lead to an encounter with a young man who attempts to rape her. She returns to her home in the suburbs—and to her mother. Esther now finds that she cannot sleep or read or write for days on end, and her doctor refers her to a psychiatrist, a handsome young man called Dr Gordon, who interviews her on only two occasions, a week apart.

During the second interview, Dr Gordon asks to speak with Esther's mother without Esther present. He decides that she should be subjected to ECT. Plath's description of ECT—administered without anaesthetic—is coldly matter-of-fact, and all the more disturbing for that. 'Dr Gordon was fitting two metal plates on either side of my head. He buckled them into place with a strap that dented my forehead and gave me a wire to bite [...] [S]omething bent down and took hold of me and shook me like the end of the world [...] [A] great jolt drubbed me till I thought my bones would break.' Esther frankly compares ECT to receiving a severe accidental electric shock when trying to move a faulty electric floor lamp as a young girl, succinctly stripping the treatment of its psychiatric mystique—except, of course, that during the accident she received the electric shock to her hands, not to her brain.

Dr Gordon tells Esther's mother: 'A few more shock treatments, Mrs Greenwood, and I think you'll notice a wonderful improvement.' But fortunately, Esther receives the ECT as an outpatient and is driven home by her mother on the same day, and so she is in a position to refuse further treatments—a decision that her mother appears to accept because she does not want her daughter to be 'Like those awful people. Those awful dead people at the hospital'.

Anyone who has read the preceding chapters will not be surprised to learn that Esther's/Sylvia's depression simply got worse. Esther takes an overdose and finds herself in another psychiatric hospital, and is eventually treated by Dr Nolan/Ruth Beuscher, who promises that she will not be subjected to ECT again, but breaks her word, despite the fact that Esther remarks: 'If anyone does that to me again I'll kill myself.' However, Esther finds ECT given under anaesthetic less traumatic than her earlier treatment.

Since Dr Nolan is 'pleased' when Esther says she hates her mother, thus starting her on the road to recovery by giving her permission to accept her real feelings, as well as sexually liberating Esther by allowing her to have a diaphragm fitted, the use of ECT seems strangely gratuitous and superfluous. We may speculate that ECT reinforced the role of Nolan/Beuscher as permanent authority figure and a surrogate mother who could act as a punitive parent when she thought it necessary.

McLean's Hospital does not seem to have been entirely enlightened or ahead of its time, as we see from Esther's chilling account of her fellow patient, a young woman called Valerie, who asks Esther to look at her scars, 'two pale marks, one on either side of her forehead, as if at some time she had started to sprout horns, but cut them off [...] "I've had a lobotomy." [...] I looked at Valerie in awe, appreciating for the first time her perpetual marble calm [...] "What will you do when you get out?" [Esther asks] "Oh, I'm not leaving," Valerie laughed. "I like it here."'. The outcome of the operation varied, turning some patients into vegetables, whether deliberately or by accident, and making others—like Valerie—perform better 'in a structured situation', as one lobotomy surgeon put it, a situation in which many were to spend their lives, as we have seen earlier. Esther, however, is destined to leave the hospital, and the book ends with her final interview with the doctors before her departure.

Unlike Hemingway, Sylvia Plath's capacity to write was not destroyed by ECT, and she was to go on to marry the British poet Ted Hughes, to move to Britain, and to write the stunning and much revered poems of the collection *Ariel* towards the end of her life. ECT ten years before her death and the antidepressant tranylcypromine—prescribed for her in the last days of her life—did nothing to prevent the return of her depression or to alleviate it. She killed herself with gas on February 10 1963 at the age of thirty. Dr Ruth Beuscher later became disillusioned with psychiatry, studied theology, and was ordained.

Faces in the Water (1961) and *An Angel at My Table* (1984) by Janet Frame

At the time of her death, the New Zealand author Janet Frame (1924–2004) was one of the most highly regarded writers in the English-speaking world. Her massive *An Autobiography*, originally published in three volumes and later republished under the original title of the second volume, *An Angel at My Table,* is one of the best examples of autobiography as major literature. Her earlier novel, *Faces in the Water,* explores Frame's own years in mental hospitals, from 1945 to 1954, in closer and more vivid detail.

We see once again, in the case of these books, that the distinction between novel and autobiography is a rather artificial one. *An Angel at My Table* is very precise on the background reasons for Janet Frame's prolonged ordeal at the hands of the psychiatric establishment of her country, while *Faces in the Water* conveys the terrifying texture of that experience. It should be added that the autobiography in particular is a wonderful portrait of New Zealand—a country that was regarded as having no literature or distinctive culture well into Frame's lifetime—and the account of the young Janet's excitement at discovering that her country *did have* a literature goes hand in hand with the pain and humiliation of her repeated confinement in mental institutions.

The book contributes enormously to New Zealand's independent cultural identity while recording its growth. For readers outside New Zealand there is an added irony and poignancy in the account of the sufferings of Janet Frame and her fellow patients: this is the country that has traditionally been regarded as most like Britain, displaying a British-style tolerance and respect for law and the rights of the individual, and also enacting seemingly exemplary policies of racial integration (the New Zealand Prime Minister Keith Holyoake was a fierce opponent of apartheid South Africa and of Ian Smith's Rhodesia). And yet —as we have seen in the earlier chapter on the spread of the use of ECT and lobotomy in the 1940s and 1950s—there is no reason to suppose that an account of years spent in British mental hospitals at that time would be any less grim. It was just that no writer of Janet Frame's stature endured the decade following the Second World War in British mental institutions and survived to publish an account of that experience.

In 1945, at the age of twenty-one, Janet Frame found that she could no longer face continuing as a painfully shy student at the teacher training college in Dunedin, New Zealand, at which she had arrived earlier that year after leaving her home and family. She took three weeks sick leave, and when this period of reprieve was over she panicked and took an overdose of aspirins, intending to kill herself. Judging by the symptoms she describes, she came close to succeeding—aspirin is almost as deadly as paracetamol in high doses.

When she realised that she would not die, Frame experienced a sense of relief and joy, as often happens with failed suicide attempts. This kind of desperate behaviour is extremely common in unprepared young adults trying to cope with the wider world, both today and in earlier decades. Fortunate young people receive compassion, reassurance and a chance to rest, and then move on. Janet Frame was not so fortunate, beginning instead upon a downward spiralling path of suffering and oppressive treatment at the hands of a society intent on interfering in her life.

She found a job washing dishes in a student canteen, but continued to submit work to the local university at which she had been following courses simultaneously with training as a teacher. Frame handed in a condensed autobiography—ironically as part of her psychology course—which she concluded with a description of her attempted suicide, and when this was read by a young psychology lecturer called John Forrest, she was 'invited' to take a rest at the Dunedin hospital.

After three weeks of observation in the psychiatric ward, the young Janet was confronted by her mother who had arrived to take her home. Janet had certainly found training as a teacher too much for her, but going home was an even more dreadful prospect, not a refuge. She screamed at her mother and refused to accompany her, supposing that she would soon be discharged from hospital and could find a job in Dunedin while she continued her university studies, and never return to teaching. Instead, she was committed to Seacliff, the mental hospital that had loomed in the landscape throughout her life (this is the consistent characteristic of mental hospitals—surely not an accidental one—as with Cefn Coed hospital in the Swansea area in South Wales). Frame adds a comment that might be repeated in varying forms by those labelled as mentally ill the world over and across the decades:

No one thought to ask me why I had screamed at my mother, no one asked me what my plans were for the future. I became an instant third person, or even personless, as in the official note about my mother's visit (reported to me many years later), 'Refused to leave hospital'.

The young writer—already published in a prestigious and very exclusive national magazine—was now a committed mental patient. The six weeks that Janet Frame spent in Seacliff changed her for life, impressing upon her the division between 'ordinary' people and the 'secret' people confined in mental hospitals, making her think of herself as one of the secret people, so that she increasingly used the words 'we' and 'us' and 'our'.

This tragic sense of fellowship has also been felt by other individuals who have gone through extraordinary experiences, such as frontline soldiers, who return to the everyday world with the conviction that 'ordinary' people can never understand them. Ernest Hemingway, a victim of ECT in the last years of his life, brilliantly depicts this condition in *Soldier's Home*, one of his early short stories; and ex-prisoners of the Soviet Gulag had a saying: *Only those who have eaten from the same bowl can understand us*.

The sheer extent of the degradation and dehumanisation that Frame witnessed made an indelible mark on her mind. Sadly for herself, but perhaps fortunately for literature and for the growth of human understanding, Janet Frame was to return to confinement in mental hospitals for most of the next nine years. She was diagnosed as suffering from schizophrenia after her first stay in Seacliff, a label that naturally stuck to her, although the diagnosis had been made 'without even talking at length to me or trying to know me or even submitting me to the standard tests which are available to psychiatrists'.

Faces in the Water is concerned with evoking the experience of long term incarceration in a mental hospital rather than with the sequence of events that lead to it. We are shown that Istina Mavet, the heroine of the novel, is intensely sensitive, vulnerable, and imaginative, and that she has vivid and distressing feelings of unreality and loss of identity. However, Istina's mental experiences (and Janet Frame's) are no more extreme than those of many readers of the novel or those of many people around us. Fortunate individuals escape the scrutiny of society. Readers of the novel will notice that the prose style is lushly poetical, sometimes to excess, and at other times the writing has a cold, grey precision.

Apart from literary considerations, however, what are we to make of this almost relentless account of hideous and unnecessary suffering? This is the world created by men like William Grey Walter of the Burden Institute in Bristol and George W. Mackay of Rampton State Institution (conventional psychiatry brought forth similar individuals in all Western industrialised societies, of course), and before them Moniz, Cerletti, and Walter Freeman. It is a world in which those who suffer from fear and sadness or a feeling of being different are subjected to more and more suffering, confidently and mercilessly, through the ignorance and arrogance of those who are appointed to run the institutions in which the 'secret' people are confined. The conditions described are in many ways worse than those that existed in Victorian asylums, and yet this is New Zealand in the years just after the defeat of Hitler and Nazism.

We are shown conditions in the mental hospital in which Istina is confined in the second chapter, finding her waking in dread in the morning to face ECT, which is used openly and with hardly an effort at pretence as a punishment and a threat by the hospital staff: 'If you don't take care you'll be for treatment tomorrow.'

Those patients who are selected to undergo ECT are informed on the day and chosen on a seemingly arbitrary and capricious basis: 'You're for treatment. No breakfast for you. Keep on your nightgown and dressing gown and take your teeth out.' Those who were not chosen on any given day had to keep themselves under control in case their elation and relief showed to the point where they might be judged unstable and liable to be given emergency treatment. Patients undergoing treatment were not given breakfast because this might cause them to vomit during the convulsions and choke or suffocate on their vomit, and this precaution became just as essential when 'modified' ECT under anaesthetic began to be used.

From Ken Kesey to Sylvia Plath to Janet Frame, and on to the psychiatric hospitals of our own day, the dreaded words 'No breakfast for you today' became synonymous with the ordeal of ECT. Some patients faced with ECT try to grab food from the other patients or vainly attempt to break out of the locked ward. There is a visit to the doorless lavatories where the patients must relieve themselves while being watched by a nurse. Even the very famous did not escape the routine degradation of hospitals in the 1950s and 1960s, including Marilyn Monroe who was faced with a doorless lavatory, locked doors, and an observation window in the door of her room when she was admitted to the Payne Whitney Psychiatric Clinic in New York in early 1961, before being rescued through the immense influence of her ex-husband Joe DiMaggio.[3] Unlike Hemingway, Marilyn Monroe escaped being subjected to ECT.

In *Faces in the Water*, the unfortunate patients sit on hard chairs at nine in the morning, having their temples rubbed with methylated spirits to increase the shock, and soon afterwards hearing the sounds of other patients convulsing or emerging into consciousness moaning and weeping: 'the treatment [...] leaves you alone and blind in a nothingness of being and you try to fumble your way like a newborn animal to the flowing of first comforts; then you wake, small and frightened, and the tears keep falling in a grief that you cannot name.'

The patients draw the explicit connection between their fear of ECT and death in the electric chair, finding also that there is no end to their dread: once they regain consciousness the anxiety begins again. Will they be 'for treatment' tomorrow? Anything can lead to being labelled 'uncooperative' and being 'put down for treatment tomorrow', including trying to speak to the doctor on his cursory rounds. ECT is applied to produce the

---

[3] Gloria Steinem, *Marilyn*, London, 1987; and James Spada and George Zeno, *Monroe*, London, 1982.

'earnest dedication to "fit in"; you learned not to cry in company but to smile and pronounce yourself pleased'.

Istina, like Janet Frame, is eventually allowed home on probation and later accepts an invitation to stay with her sister and brother-in-law in northern New Zealand, the warmest — indeed semi-tropical — part of the country, where she is confined to another mental hospital for no better reason (one is tempted to say 'for no worse crime') than experiencing feelings of unreality, dislocation, terror, and loss of identity. More ECT follows in a special ward in which 'I heard the familiar calamitous despairing cry of a patient undergoing ECT and snorting noises in the room next door, and the sound of something being wheeled along the corridor to my room'.

The patients are told — as people continue to be told today, and as psychiatric professionals continue to tell themselves — that the treatment is for their own good. '"For your own good" is a persuasive argument that will eventually make man agree to his own destruction', Istina reflects before finding that her terror continues to mount, so that she is eventually transferred to a ward for people who are considered to be more serious cases. 'The squalor and inhumanity were almost indescribable.' Janet Frame recalls of this time in her life, making the startling admission that she omitted much from *Faces in the Water* 'because I did not want a record by a former patient to appear to be over-dramatic'. And yet in the wards known as Park House, 'human beings became or were quickly transformed into living as animals'. When she was eventually transferred back to the admission ward, 'thin, with sores and a discharging ear', she was brought six free copies of her book, *The Lagoon and Other Stories,* just published in New Zealand by The Caxton Press. It is one of the strangest aspects of Frame's life — and one of its greatest ironies — that literary success kept pace with terrible subjugation as one of the 'secret' people.

Istina is released, as Janet Frame was, from the mental hospital 'up north' and returns to her family home, from which she is sent again to her first mental hospital, called Cliffhaven in the novel, having once again experienced extreme, hallucinatory panic and dislocation of reality, just as Frame returned to Seacliff after her mother suffered a heart attack.

Istina, like Janet Frame, is soon removed to the back ward to become one of 'the forgotten people'. One of the nurses in *Faces in the Water* is called Sister Bridge—names are almost as important in this book as they are in *One Flew Over the Cuckoo's Nest*—a woman who has achieved a sympathetic rapport with many of the patients. However, this Bridge Over Troubled Water turns out to be a treacherous one. When she catches Istina *observing* her being kind to the patients, Sister Bridge is filled with resentment and does everything she can to oppress and humiliate Istina.

The tyrannous Matron Glass is as dreary a servant of the system as Kesey's Miss Ratched, but a far more fragile one: 'Seeing her without her uniform one knew that the uniform and veil were a desperate protection for her [...] [S]he seemed to be stripped of all her power, so much so that she seemed to have an air of helplessness and pathos.'

These psychological insights, directed as they are towards the *oppressors*, go beyond Ken Kesey and demonstrate a superior literary power. The description of the patients who have undergone lobotomies and become more docile, but who are now indifferent to soiling themselves while being enthusiastically 'retrained' for a short time by nurses who quickly lose interest in them, is as chilling as anything in Kesey's novel.

Janet Frame's mother had signed her consent for her daughter to undergo a lobotomy/leucotomy, and one of the doctors explained that 'it would be good for me' and 'I would be out of hospital in no time'. Janet's name was added to the list of those to be lobotomised—the new convenience treatment—that hung in the ward office. Frame's writing saved her. The superintendent of the hospital, Dr Blake Palmer, visited the ward with a newspaper announcing that Janet Frame had been given the Hubert Church Award for the best prose for her book *The Lagoon*, and therefore he countermanded the leucotomy. A friend of Janet's called Nola, who had not won a prize or appeared in a newspaper, was given a leucotomy and remained in hospital.

Janet Frame was finally discharged from hospital, 'having received over two hundred applications of unmodified ECT, each the equivalent, in degree of fear, to an execution [...] [H]aving been subjected to proposals to have myself changed, by a physical operation, into a more acceptable, amenable, normal person, I arrived home [...] with the conviction at last that I was officially a non-person'. As we read these words, we should reflect that during Frame's time in mental hospitals, in the year 1949, Orwell's novel *Nineteen Eighty-Four* was published. The years of Western condemnation of the abuse of psychiatry in the Soviet Union lay decades ahead, and Walter Reich was to write of that abuse: 'Those Soviet psychiatrists really *saw* the patients as schizophrenic [...] *the system created a category, first on paper, and then with training, in the minds of Soviet psychiatrists* [...]'.[4] We may be sure that the psychiatrists responsible for diagnosing Janet Frame as schizophrenic—as well as psychiatrists throughout the Western world—would strenuously deny that Reich's description also applies to them.

(A highly praised film version of *An Angel at My Table* was directed by Jane Campion. I have omitted it from discussion here for reasons of space.)

Girl, Interrupted
by Susanna Kaysen (1993)

Susanna Kaysen's book does not contain the portrayal of relentless cruelty and suffering that is found in Janet Frame's autobiography and novel, and coming to it straight from Frame's writing, we may find a certain tone of self-indulgence—something that Kaysen acknowledges.

Susanna Kaysen was sent to McLean Hospital—where Sylvia Plath had been a patient more than a decade earlier—on April 27 1967, following an interview lasting about twenty minutes with a doctor who had never seen her before. She was

---

[4] Walter Reich, 'Psychiatric diagnosis as an ethical problem', in *Psychiatric Ethics*, edited by S. Bloch and P. Chodoff, Oxford, 1984.

seventeen. Susanna signed herself in, and thus signed away her rights, because she was given to understand that if she did not do so there would be a court order made to have her admitted. She realised in later life that no court order could have been made under US law at that time, but on that April day she believed what she was led to believe.

She was diagnosed as suicidally depressed by the doctor who spoke to her for twenty minutes, and later diagnosed as suffering from a borderline schizophrenic reaction and from Borderline Personality Disorder. Her family continued to pay very large sums for her to be treated at McLean, where she was to remain for nearly two years, presumably in preference to her incarceration in a state mental hospital.

In *Girl, Interrupted* we face the issue of a certain collusion or connivance with an oppressive system on the part of Kaysen and on the part of the other young women locked up with her and their families, the same issue that arises in *One Flew Over the Cuckoo's Nest* with regard to the fictional male patients who chose to remain in hospital. Janet Frame was far more of a clear-cut victim of cruelty and ignorance. Nevertheless, it is difficult for the reader not to like Susanna for her wit, humour, intelligence, glamour, sexuality, and—rather surprisingly—for the vitality and confidence that she possesses without altogether realising that she has it. Janet Frame, by contrast, does tend to dwell rather lugubriously on her decaying teeth, intense shyness and lack of boyfriends. A unique feature of Kaysen's book is the reproduction of documents from the 350 pages of her hospital file, obtained with the help of a lawyer, enabling her to underpin an attack on the psychiatric system that is both devastating and subtle.

The social atmosphere in America at that time is important in *Girl, Interrupted*, just as it had been in Plath's *The Bell Jar*, and Susanna speculates that the oppressive and irresponsible actions of the doctor who sent her to McLean were partly a response to the 'threatening' attitude of rebellion found among American youth in the 1960s: 'there was a strange undertow, a tug from the other world—the drifting, drugged-out, no-last-name youth universe [...] And then one of them walks into his office wearing a skirt the size of a napkin, with a mottled chin and speaking in monosyllables.'

The loss of two years of a young woman's life is, of course, a rather high price to pay in order to alleviate middle-class alarm at the upheavals in American society, but Kaysen, like Frame, is making an honest attempt to see those who run the system as trapped by society and by the system itself. The doctor stands for authority and legitimacy, and Susanna realises how reluctant many of her readers would be to believe her account of events that occurred when she was seventeen and depressed—most of all being sent to McLean after an interview lasting only twenty minutes—without the reproduction of the hospital's Admission Note in her text.

She was admitted to a world in which the loss of freedom was severe, despite McLean's good reputation, the cost of being there, and the famous Americans who had been treated there. Susanna found herself in a ward of 'medium security', but this meant 'double-locked doors, our steel-mesh window screens, our kitchen stocked with plastic knives and locked unless a nurse was with us, our bathroom doors that didn't lock'. The mad logic of McLean is quite as crazy as the hospital of Kesey's novel and the institutions in which Janet Frame was confined: it deemed these restrictions appropriate for a group of very unhappy young women whose worst crimes were suicide attempts, in a few cases using drugs, and a general refusal or inability to fit into society.

One of Kaysen's fellow patients, a young woman called Alice, 'exploded like a volcano [...] yelling and crashing came out of the seclusion room [...] Her face was puffy from crying and bashing around'. Alice does no worse than this—no injuries inflicted on staff or other patients, no murder committed, but she is taken to a ward of 'maximum security' in which 'the rooms were not really rooms. They were cells. [...] There wasn't anything in them except bare mattresses with people on them [...] [T]he windows were tiny, high, chicken-wire-enforced, security-screened, barred windows. Most of the doors to the rooms were open, so as we walked down the hall to see Alice, we could see other people lying on their mattresses. Some were naked'.

Fortunately, Susanna is not subjected to ECT, but another young woman called Cynthia undergoes it for six months: 'crying after electroshock ("I'm not sad," she explained to me, "but I can't help crying.").' We may recall Janet Frame's description of regaining consciousness after ECT, 'then you wake, small and frightened, and the tears keep falling in a grief that you cannot name'. There is indeed a remarkable continuity, and remarkable similarities, in the descriptions of mental hospital experiences considered in this chapter. Kaysen and all her fellow patients are routinely — almost capriciously — subjected to sedation: 'Thorazine, Stelazine, Mellaril, Librium, Valium: the therapists' friends. The resident could put us on that stuff too [...] "You're doing so well," the resident would say. That was because those things knocked the heart out of us.'

One chapter is entitled '1968', evoking the atmosphere of the times, including the television images of protest and upheaval and dissent that were greeted with cheers by the patients, despite the fact that these patients were locked into a dangerous collusion with the hospital system; having lost 'our privacy, our liberty, our dignity' they were protected from the real world — like the patients around Kesey's McMurphy — by the hospital that confined and humiliated them. And sometimes this arrangement could be turned on its head, as in the case of the young woman called Torrey, who is drugged with chlorpromazine to make her compliant when being sent out of the hospital and back to the family she hates.

Susanna Kaysen quotes the American textbook *Diagnostic and Statistical Manual of Mental Disorders* (3rd edition, 1987), which gives a definition of the condition called Borderline Personality Disorder from which she was supposedly suffering:

> An essential feature of this disorder is a pervasive pattern of instability of self-image, interpersonal relationships, and mood, beginning in early adulthood and present in a variety of contexts. A marked and persistent identity disturbance is almost

invariably present. This is often pervasive, and is manifested by uncertainty about several life issues, such as self-image, sexual orientation, long-term goals or career choice, types of friends or lovers to have, and which values to adopt.

Kaysen admits that this is a fairly accurate description of herself at the time she was sent to hospital. Her 'illness' consisted of having enthusiasm only for literature and 'boyfriends by the barrelful', as well as an aversion to the demands of her parents, the educational system, and society in general, which amounted to a complete inability to accommodate those demands. This tedious and repetitive passage from the *Diagnostic and Statistical Manual* is also a fairly accurate description of a great many adolescents and young adults, but it is in no way a description of an illness, unless being young is defined as an illness, which many psychiatrists might like to do. Susanna Kaysen, like Janet Frame, became an author, insisting that she was accepted on her own terms and making 'a life out of boyfriends and literature'.

The 1999 film entitled *Girl, Interrupted,* starring Winona Ryder, Whoopi Goldberg, and Angelina Jolie, is an excellent piece of cinematic art, but it is rather far removed from the original text, almost an analogy rather than a commentary in terms of the categories set out by the critic Geoffrey Wagner. The head nurse Valerie, played by Whoopi Goldberg, is given a substantially different character in the film, and so is the patient called Lisa, played by Angelina Jolie. The film is a *story* in a way that Susanna Kaysen's frequently plotless and non-linear narrative is not, including the clash of characters, conflict, dramatic scenes, and a final resolution of sorts. It is fair to ask whether Hollywood's need to force films into clearly defined genres allows for any film that is not a story of this kind.

Lisa becomes a McMurphy-like character—indeed the film can be described as a kind of *One Flew Over the Cuckoo's Nest II* (with women). The film is a drama of growing into adulthood and Susanna's acceptance of herself, while the book remains a thoughtful and highly intelligent set of reminiscences.

In Two Minds by David Mercer (1967) and *Family Life* (1972) written by David Mercer and directed by Ken Loach

David Mercer's superb television play *In Two Minds*, and the equally impressive film *Family Life* for which he wrote the screenplay, tell the same story, although the order in which incidents happen and the characters themselves differ significantly in each work.

In both the film and the play the central character is a young woman in her early twenties. The young woman is called Kate in the play and Janice in the film, and the story follows her breakdown into mental illness under the pressure put upon her by her parents and by the psychiatric profession—it might be more accurate to say that the story traces her destruction rather than her breakdown: this bleak and convincing tale leaves us with little hope that Kate/ Janice—any more than millions of her real life counterparts—will escape profound and permanent damage or will ever be able to live a normal life.

The film is more ambitious in that it attempts a wider attack on society in general and the conformity it demands from its members, particularly from young women. These works give a picture of the moment to moment detail and texture of the experience of breakdown that is not equalled by the other books and films considered in this chapter, and television and film is, of course, perfectly suited to following this process.

The central situation in the story is a simple one. Kate/Janice has a suffocatingly domineering mother and a father who is too ineffectual to stand up to his wife and stand up for his daughter, while Kate/Janice herself has been weakened and conditioned throughout her whole life to lack the confidence to defy her mother, and when she does assert herself she quickly succumbs to the guilt that has been instilled into her. Any attempt to be a person in her own right and to live her own life is defined as 'letting down' her parents, 'upsetting' her mother, or making her mother 'ill'.

It is important to recognise that the father is not a bad man, but he is hopelessly inhibited by the role and expectations of working-class men of his generation, a role that excluded him from actively bringing up or guiding his daughter, which he has been conditioned to see as the role of the mother. The father's natural inclinations would have made him a very different husband and father, but the habit of obedience to his wife and his sense of inferiority towards her (he could never admit to either these things, of course) has made him fit only to endorse her view of things, back her up, and occasionally boil over with rage at his daughter. When Kate/Janice was a little girl he was an affectionate and fun loving father, but he was effectively prevented from continuing in this way by his wife, and similarly his sexual life with his wife is grossly inhibited or—more probably—non-existent.

The mother is obsessed with her own fears about the dirtiness and dangers of sex, and in the film—very much like Susanna Kaysen's doctor—this obsession is fuelled partly by her fear of the upheavals of the 1960s. Kate/Janice has an older sister who has left home at seventeen and now feels little more than outright hatred for her parents, while their mother has reacted to the departure of her older daughter by tying Kate/Janice to her all the more tightly. The mother is a truly frightening and repulsive figure, but it is important to realise that she is also deeply insecure, a damaged and frightened personality who is not capable of love and therefore is driven to possess and control her daughter.

Kate's/Janice's mother strongly disapproves of her daughter's friends and boyfriends (there could be no one she would approve of), and when her daughter gets pregnant unintentionally, the mother is once again 'proved right'. The mother puts enormous pressure upon her daughter—who eventually gives in—to have an abortion, claiming all the while to hate abortion and to consider it criminal.

Mental illness, particularly the set of symptoms that were ambitiously and disastrously called 'dementia praecox' or 'schizophrenia' a century ago, often develops in late adolescence and early adulthood. Many readers of this book and many of those who have watched *In Two Minds* and *Family Life* will find the portrayal of Kate's/Janice's mother dismally familiar. Real life and David Mercer's brilliant depiction force us to ask a number of questions. Is it surprising that someone who has been subjected to the din of voices — one voice particularly — that tell her what she wants, what she feels, and who she is for years on end begins to hear hallucinatory voices? Is it surprising that someone who is subtly controlled by parental disapproval and by internalised guilt for years begins to feel that she is a robot controlled from a distance? Is it surprising that someone who is denied a life of her own and even the opportunity to think her own thoughts retreats into some inner mental state?

Kate/Janice believes at times that her mother is trying to kill her. But of course, in an important sense, her mother *is killing her*, by preventing her from living an individual life. Yet these symptoms — hallucinatory voices, passive feelings of being controlled, withdrawal, feelings of being persecuted and plotted against — are pompously and dangerously defined as evidence of an illness originating in the brain chemistry of the sufferer. Kate's/Janice's mother *is* constantly plotting against her, although she cannot admit that she is doing this.

There is a chilling scene in the television play in which Kate and her mother are shopping and Kate is about to buy a dress she really wants. Kate's mother begins by telling her daughter that she doesn't really want the dress at all, and then she retreats into saying that it is Kate's decision and that Kate must do as she wishes, but along the way she conveys that the dress is too short (and thus contaminated by the poison of sex). The mother even finally says: 'It's quite pretty, in a way. Yes', which will be her defence in case of future recriminations. The mother's disapproval is enough to stop Kate buying the dress, compelling her to tell the shop assistant that 'I don't think it's right for me'.

However, Kate has not been allowed to *think* for herself at all, instead her mother's thoughts have been thrust into her mind and used to control her, and yet psychiatrists in the story and in real life see the belief that thoughts are being projected into a patient's head as a classic symptom of 'schizophrenia'. The mother's methods of control are far more insidious — and thus infinitely more destructive—than outright physical intimidation, and we should not underestimate the effect of thousands of small incidents such as the dress buying scene that have been repeated over many years. Her husband expresses it perfectly: 'Dolly [his wife] wouldn't prevent nobody doing nothing! It's not in her nature.' Kate asks: 'Have *I* got a point of view? [...] They're jerking at me... pulling at me—with the wires. They've got these wires attached... they run inside my head, into my brain...'

A humane psychiatrist who does not use invasive physical means of treatment is an important figure in the story. He is in charge of a ward in the film and an investigating doctor in the play, and in both works he tries to build up Kate's/Janice's awareness that her 'illness' comes from being denied her own individuality and her own independent life, and in both the film and the play he is defeated. In *Family Life* his appointment at the hospital is not renewed, and in *In Two Minds* Kate simply gives up all hope before his influence can have any effect.

The fragile young woman's mind increasingly gives way after the abortion, partly because she is told repeatedly that she 'cannot cope', which is, of course, the last thing her mother wants her to be able to do. In the play Kate's sister tells her: 'I don't think you're ill at all. You're weak.' Perhaps this is true, and yet, after all, the combined power of the mother and of the psychiatric system is formidable. Some people rise above social disadvantage and racial discrimination; some people survive sexual abuse, violent relationships, and prolonged bullying at school; others are destroyed by these things. Are those who are destroyed 'weak', or simply not quite as strong?

Kate/Janice is given tranquillisers, subjected to ECT, and paraded in front of medical students as a 'case history' by a consultant psychiatrist. This hideously damaged human being will be returned to her mother's possession for the rest of her life, another victim of the failure to 'offer human understanding'.

Two Psychiatrists and a Literary Critic:
R.D. Laing, Martin Seymour-Smith, and William Sargant

The last section of this chapter pushes at the limits set out in the chapter title, but I have included it in order to fill out the picture of the part psychiatry plays in our culture. Firstly, we should glance briefly at the movement known as anti-psychiatry that arose in the 1960s, and at its most famous advocate, Ronald David Laing (1927–1989). Laing's own violent, abusive, and deeply unhappy childhood in a poor area of Glasgow, as well as his early experiences as an army psychiatrist between 1951 and 1953, shaped his outlook and approach to questions of sanity, madness, and the power wielded by psychiatrists.

Laing's first book *The Divided Self* (1960) is a work of considerable literary power, and one of the first authoritative non-fiction accounts of the way in which psychiatrists and society in general label and objectify those who suffer from mental breakdowns and crises as 'Them'. The book also attempts a philosophical—or existential—account of madness: in Laing's view schizophrenics suffer from an 'ontological insecurity', an uncertainty about their own being and existence that leads to terror and inner chaos.

The young R.D. Laing showed an extraordinary gift for empathising with those suffering from psychotic states, and there is a wonderful passage in *The Divided Self* in which he quotes a 1905 lecture on clinical psychiatry by Emil Kraepelin (1856–1926), during which a patient was paraded in front of a room full of students (just as David Mercer's Kate/Janice is exhibited by a consultant). Kraepelin sees the patient's long outburst as a series of symptoms of an illness, stating that 'he [the patient] has not given us a single piece of useful information'. The patient's admittedly bizarre and oblique monologue is very convincingly shown by Laing to be an expression of his resentment and sense of humiliation at being turned into a performing animal by Kraepelin, as well as his way of ridiculing Kraepelin (possibly expressed in convoluted terms out of fear of the consequences). Kraepelin is merely looking for pathological symptoms in his victim, while Laing sees the words of this young man as expressions of his feelings and his experiences.

Unfortunately, Laing's later work deteriorated as he fashionably described those suffering from psychosis as sane people in an insane world, so that the methods he used in an alternative refuge for patients became increasingly dangerous and irresponsible. Also, Laing's use of LSD and his legendary hard drinking seem to have pushed him further away from a compassionate appraisal of suffering and further trivialised his work. Both the American psychiatrist Peter R. Breggin and the British psychologist Richard P. Bentall have acknowledged the groundbreaking importance of Laing's early work in their books. Sadly, Laing never quite attained the clarity, responsibility, coherence, and humanity of Breggin and Bentall.

Martin Seymour-Smith (1928–1998) was an extraordinarily prolific literary critic and biographer of great richness of mind, integrity, and intellectual independence. He also pronounced confidently (perhaps dogmatically) on psychiatry and mental illness, especially in his later work.

The first edition of Seymour-Smith's huge book *Guide to Modern World Literature* (1973) does not include any discussion of mental illness as such (that is, other than the problems of individual writers), but the revised and expanded *Guide* (1985) devotes a substantial part of the long introduction to this subject, including an attack on R.D. Laing, who — according to Seymour-Smith — 'just likes sick and destructive people, whom he can then call sane by definition'. There is no acknowledgement of the liberating and perceptive quality of Laing's early work, and instead we are told that Laing's ideas are 'so misguided as to be positively wicked […] and very unkind. The literature which has been modelled on his ideas is junk […] It is an insult to the human spirit, and a cruel lie'. This is strong stuff by any standards, although Seymour-Smith was always pugnacious in his language.

Laing and mental illness keep cropping up in the 1985 *Guide* in a way that does not occur in the 1973 version. In the *Guide's* section on Doris Lessing (who was later to win the Nobel Prize for Literature 2007, but is not very highly regarded by Seymour-Smith), Laing is called a 'wily little pasteboard mage'. Mental illness, confident statements on its nature and treatment, and R.D. Laing particularly, seem to have become distinct preoccupations in Seymour-Smith's later work, although we must presumably wait for a biography of this highly gifted man before we have an explanation of these preoccupations.

In the *Guide's* introduction we find an approving reference to antipsychotic drugs: 'really the first effective one was chlorpromazine (largactil) [sic] available from the early Fifties.' The misspelling of the drug's name and the spelling of its trade name with a lower case first letter are oddly disturbing in a book by a writer who clearly believes he has considerable medical expertise. Seymour-Smith says nothing of the way in which chlorpromazine acts according to psychiatrists, and he does not mention any of its serious side effects. It would be easier to trust Seymour-Smith's competence in this field if some of his other statements were more historically accurate and consistent.

We are told in the 1985 *Guide* that Ernest Hemingway 'shot himself in a fit of depression for which he preferred not to be treated', although the truth is that Hemingway *did allow himself to be treated for depression*, and lost his memory after being subjected to ECT, thus further diminishing his will to live. Seymour-Smith scorns a critic who described Sylvia Plath as a schizophrenic, informing us that the critic was 'no doctor'. (And yet doctors, not literary critics, diagnosed Janet Frame as suffering from schizophrenia and Susanna Kaysen as suffering from a borderline schizophrenic reaction and Borderline Personality Disorder!)

There is a section on the poet Ivor Gurney who spent the last years of his life in mental institutions 'at a time when there was virtually no treatment, except kindness, for any severe mental disturbance'. (We may feel tempted to say that it is a great pity that this treatment has not been more widely used — in the past and today.)

In Seymour-Smith's eyes David Mercer suffers from guilt by association with the ideas of R.D. Laing (again), ignoring the fact that the story told in *Family Life* and *In Two Minds* is entirely convincing in itself and does not depend on the ideas of Laing or anyone else. It may be significant that a literary critic of such great gifts falls below his usual high standards at the very points at which he is to some extent justifying conventional psychiatry.

Martin Seymour-Smith also wrote a biography of his close friend, the poet Robert Graves, *Robert Graves: His Life and Work* (revised edition 1995), and in it we find the following surprising statement regarding the year 1956: 'he [Graves] polished [...] *Battle for the Mind*, to which he contributed the chapter about brainwashing in ancient times, for its author, the mad psychiatrist Dr William Sargant (he took a third of the proceeds, Sargant two-thirds).' It is the career of William Sargant (1907–1988) that we must examine in the last part of this section. A superb radio documentary on Sargant called *Revealing the Mind Bender General* was made by the writer and broadcaster James Maw and broadcast in 2009 and 2010.[5] I am most indebted to Mr Maw's work, as anyone striving to understand William Sargant must be.

St Thomas's Hospital at which Sargant became head of the Department of Psychological Medicine in 1948 stands near to the Ministry of Defence and the headquarters of MI6. Sargant ran Ward Five of the hospital through the 1960s and 1970s, where patients were subjected to his Deep Sleep Treatment in what was called the Sleep Room. Two of these patients, Anne White and a woman who wished to be known only as June, have recalled their experiences in the Sleep Room. June described Sargant as a handsome, leonine man who talked at his patients but did not listen to them. Anne was admitted in the early 1970s suffering from post-natal depression, and she was soon to be subjected to Sargant's continuous narcosis, rendered unconscious by drugs for six weeks, during which she was regularly given ECT, having been fed periodically in a semi-conscious state.

---

[5] *Revealing the Mind Bender General* by James Maw, BBC Radio 4, broadcast April 1 2009 and March 17 2010 (http://www.jamesmaw.co.uk, last accessed on March 17 2011)

Ironically, like the lobotomist Walter Freeman, Sargant also suffered from depression at times throughout his life. In 1940, he had established a psychiatric unit at Belmont, near Sutton, at which he performed psychological experiments on soldiers evacuated from Dunkirk, using 'abreaction' and instilling terror by forcing traumatised servicemen to relive their experiences for allegedly therapeutic purposes. The politician and former Labour cabinet minister Lord David Owen worked with Sargant and still defends him. When Sargant published an article on his methods in *The Lancet* in 1940, he was told by the Ministry of Defence not to publish any more material on the subject. Clearly, people in high levels of government had interests of their own in this kind of work and considered it too sensitive to be publicised. Lord Owen remarked: 'I wouldn't be a bit surprised if he [Sargant] was speaking to people on the fringe of brainwashing.'

Sargant stated in his own autobiography that he had been 'privy to secrets at the highest level'. He may have been the psychiatrist in charge of experiments on selected victims using LSD at the Porton Down Psychiatric Unit in 1953, although this has not been proved. However, he subjected ordinary patients like Anne White and June to his methods, combining continuous narcosis and frequent ECT, while he was working for the National Health Service.

June, who had been trained as a nurse, recognised one of the substances given to her as a truth drug, sodium pentothal or Sodium Amytal, which was administered during periods of wakefulness in the weeks she was kept asleep. She also woke up after ECT in 'complete and utter terror', not even remembering her name. Like Janet Frame, June could not foresee any end to her incarceration.

Anne was given large doses of chlorpromazine as well as ECT, and had large parts of her memory wiped clean, and she recalls that 'there was no informed consent at all' to any of this. Dr Malcolm Lader, now Professor of Clinical Psychopharmacology, was horrified at what he saw when he visited Sargant's

Ward Five, not least because of the lack of any attempt to assess the treatment given.

Methods that were similar to Sargant's were being used by D. Ewen Cameron in Canada and Harry Bailey in Australia. Cameron—who was partly funded by the CIA because of their interest in brainwashing—caused permanent damage to more than fifty patients, and Harry Bailey caused the deaths of between twenty and twenty-five of his patients. Sargant stated that as a result of 679 treatments carried out on 484 of his patients, four of them had died. However, he gave no names or dates for these deaths, and—rather conveniently for the medical establishment—records were not kept by St Thomas's Hospital. He remarked in his last interview: 'I suppose this horrifies people today.'

No compensation or damages have ever been paid to Sargant's victims. Michael Neve of The Wellcome Trust Centre for the History of Medicine describes Sargant's programme as 'mercilessly anti-psychotherapeutic'.[6] In an article of his own written in 1961 Sargant was supremely confident, declaring that whereas other, non-invasive therapies had been 'fully explored', physical treatments were in 'relative infancy'.[7] This was written after nearly three decades of insulin coma therapy, lobotomy, and ECT, and as Michael Neve comments 'his remark bears some pondering'.

How could a man of the intelligence of the poet Robert Graves have failed to see that Sargant's attitudes and approach were sinister and dangerous, and so allow himself to collaborate with such a man for profit? Such actions hardly seem to be reconcilable with common decency, a quality that Martin Seymour-Smith refers to frequently, just as Orwell did. It is not surprising that a man like Dr Joseph Mengele—who experimented on twins and handicapped people at Auschwitz—

---

[6] Michael Neve, 'A commentary on the history of social psychiatry and psychotherapy in twentieth-century Germany, Holland and Britain', *Medical History*, 48: 407–412, 2004.

[7] William Sargant, 'The treatment prognosis for functional psychoses in Great Britain', *American Journal of Psychiatry*, 1961 (*The Sargant Papers, Archives and Manuscripts*, Wellcome Library, London).

prospered in Nazi Germany, but it is deeply shocking to discover that men like William Sargant prosper in our own society. What gives some educated, affluent and powerful men their incredible enthusiasm and zeal for cruelty? Why is it that a democratic society is unable to restrain them?

Chapter Five

Informed Consent

This is not a book of personal reminiscences, but I would like to expand somewhat on the autobiographical details in the first chapter by giving some personal impressions of the psychiatric profession, although I may disappoint those readers who have hoped that they are reading an account by a detached expert.

I have never been subjected to ECT or detained behind locked doors against my will, so that my experiences have been —mercifully—very limited. Nevertheless, some details may be worth recounting. I began to suffer from depression with some morbid obsessional symptoms at the age of seventeen, and I was distressed enough to go to my GP, who referred me to a consultant psychiatrist. I remember this psychiatrist very well— let's call him Dr Smith—a large, charismatic, grey-haired man in a crumpled suit, possessing considerable charm and *presence*, so that he seemed to exert a gravitational pull in any room he entered. I later learned that he had undergone terrible ordeals and had been through distinguished adventures in the Second World War.

The late summer and autumn of 1974 were overcast and oppressive seasons in the place in which I lived, in the world generally, and in the landscape of my own emotions, but I retained my interest in current events, which always seemed to me as important as the details of my own life—something that kept me saner than I realised at that time. The Russian writer Alexander Solzhenitsyn had been expelled from the Soviet Union in the February of that year, the philosopher and scientist Jacob Bronowski died unexpectedly at the height of his powers in the August, less than two weeks after the resignation of President Richard Nixon in disgrace. These were depressing times! I do not recall that I ever talked to Dr Smith about world affairs, but I saw him about five times over a period of six months.

I was prescribed diazepam, a sleeping pill called nitrazepam, and a tricyclic antidepressant called clomipramine, and later, a drug called Triptafen, a combination of the tricyclic antidepressant amitriptyline and perphenazine, a neuroleptic related to chlorpromazine. None of these chemicals made me feel better, but I trusted Dr Smith and believed that he knew what he was doing, after all, one of his frequently repeated remarks was 'We only have to find the right drug'.

After about six months, he suggested that I allowed myself to be admitted to hospital on a voluntary basis, assuring me that it would be much easier to 'find the right drug' under hospital conditions. I gave serious consideration to this suggestion and then decided against it, writing a letter to Dr Smith to inform him of my decision. I may have seen him on one or two further occasions, but he never pressed the matter of my going into hospital.

It is at the point at which this psychiatrist suggested that I should go into hospital that my story becomes strikingly similar to the accounts of depression in adolescence and early adulthood found in the books we considered in the last chapter. I was simply more fortunate than others.

If I had been admitted to Swansea's Cefn Coed hospital I would have been defined as a young man already suffering from depression for several months, having failed to respond to antidepressants, and I would have been given even more powerful antidepressants and neuroleptics as a matter of course. These drugs make people more compliant and easier to control. Further, a mental hospital is a strange and sometimes threatening environment, and above all it is a place in which patients are dependent upon authority figures. I was to meet about twenty of Dr Smith's patients and former patients a decade after my own encounters with him, and I learned that he very much favoured ECT, so that one of his ex-patients even joked that he was paid commission on every ECT session by the national electricity provider.

Would he have told me that I should have ECT? I can picture myself as a young man just turned eighteen, scared, isolated, my concentration and awareness blunted by drugs that had also rendered me less able to assert myself, lacking words or arguments to use against this powerful, charismatic man (no doubt backed up by a glamorous nurse or two) who seemed to want to help me. And if I had refused? How easy it would have been to call in another psychiatrist and have my status changed to that of a detained patient, so that I could then have been subjected to ECT without my consent.

Dr Smith was a formidable man, and it is not easy to imagine another doctor disagreeing with his diagnosis, even if that doctor felt there was any reason to disagree. Perhaps we should also recall the cautionary words of the Soviet dissident Andrei Amalrik, quoted in Chapter 1, 'one psychiatrist will always have more faith in the words of another psychiatrist than of a patient'. I would probably have been sent home after ECT with large areas of my memory erased, quite possibly becoming one of the 'revolving door' patients who succumb to depression again and again and find themselves back in hospital, compelled to undergo more ECT. I prided myself upon my independence of mind and my refusal to conform, and yet how easily I might have become another victim, another statistic! Fortunately for me, however, none of this happened, and I gave up taking antidepressants — but not the highly addictive diazepam (Valium) — when my depression cleared up spontaneously.

Sadly, this was not quite the end of my experience of mental disturbance and of the psychiatric profession. I developed severe anxiety for a short time at the age of nineteen, so that I was trembling constantly, starting at every sound, and I trembled even more when one GP told me confidently — almost cheerfully — that I was suffering from schizophrenia. (I had never heard of Janet Frame in those days, and so I did not know that I was in distinguished and honourable company.)

I saw another psychiatrist—let us call him Dr Jones—though only on two occasions. Dr Jones was spectacularly uninterested in my condition, and he was also a very strange man. It is said that those who suffer from psychotic illnesses are often withdrawn, emotionally flat, and unable to communicate with others, speaking in monosyllables—and this very precisely describes Dr Jones. He prescribed me lorazepam—a more powerful and more addictive version of diazepam—and chlorpromazine, although only for a short time.

The trouble arose when my regular GP glanced at my notes and continued to prescribe me chlorpromazine for the next five years—this neuroleptic can cause irreversible tardive dyskinesia after only a short time—but I knew no better, and when my severe anxiety cleared up I attributed my recovery to the medication. Prescribing chlorpromazine for anxiety for years on end would still be astonishingly irresponsible even if there was any serious scientific basis for its use in psychotic illness.

I was to have a third and—thankfully—final encounter with the psychiatric world when I continuously drank myself into unconsciousness in the autumn of 1982, just before my twenty-sixth birthday. Well, I was hardly unique among young men of that age in drinking excessively and dangerously, but I went further than most and woke with a raging thirst in Ward F of Cefn Coed hospital. The standard treatment for those who abused alcohol was to take away their clothes (and of course deprive them of alcohol) and let them 'dry out', alleviating the agonising process of acute alcoholic withdrawal with diazepam and chlormethiazole.

The rules are changed for alcohol abusers, however: I was not really a psychiatric patient, and there was nothing preventing me from demanding my clothes and leaving in order to start drinking again. No one would—or could—have invoked the Mental Health Act in order to have me detained and treated against my will, and I knew it. I merely realised that I had come close to killing myself with alcohol and decided that I ought to give myself a breathing space and stop drinking. When the dreadful symptoms of alcoholic withdrawal passed off I began to observe my surroundings with some interest, and talk to the other patients.

The things I saw and heard in Ward F—reinforced by getting to know many people labelled mentally ill in the years that followed—would in themselves provide the material for a substantial book. Several patients would obviously never leave that hospital, and several more had been in and out of hospital for years. It gradually became clear to me that many patients were disabled far more by drugs and ECT than by any original illness, although I did not have the technical information at that time to enable me to understand why this was so.

One image stands out in my mind. A woman aged about sixty was pacing up and down in the corridor of the ward, her face stricken by some intolerable anguish, and then a nurse called out to her from the nurses' office in a bored and casual voice that could be heard by everyone around. 'Sandra! The doctor wants you to have ECT!' The nurse did not even stand up or put down the cup of tea she was drinking.

In the following year I realised that—like millions of others —I was heavily addicted to the lorazepam prescribed for me, and I spent eight terrifying months slowly reducing my intake of the drug and finally gave it up after prolonged withdrawal symptoms that resembled a mental and physical illness. I felt that I wanted to give something back to life in return for my own good fortune, and so I worked for a drug advice unit based in the community. The project was new, and after some basic training we were left to get on with things. I met nearly a hundred people addicted to prescribed drugs over the next two years, and many of them had also received other kinds of psychiatric treatment, including ECT. Some years later, I wrote a piece of fiction about ECT based on the composite experience of several people. The piece was published in the magazine *Social Care Education* (Number 11, autumn 1991). I include it here.

Informed Consent

After the first ten days in hospital, she was brought to Dr Gibson. For the first few minutes Dr Gibson stared at her in silence, then asked a few routine medical questions and wrote down the answers. Then the phone rang. Dr Gibson picked it up and without looking at her she waved her hand at Marilyn to indicate that she should leave the office until the call was finished. She had to do this several times before Marilyn realised what she meant and got up and went outside. When Dr Gibson brought her back, she began questioning Marilyn about the state she had been in since the birth of her baby. She seemed unsatisfied with the answers Marilyn gave her and kept on asking questions. Marilyn kept thinking how Dr Gibson's mouth, with the deep lines running from it across the jaw, reminded her of a statue she had seen in childhood and had disliked. At last she became confused and began to sob.

'My baby — my baby', she kept repeating, then suddenly she screamed at Dr Gibson, 'Have you got children?'

'No, Mrs Pearce.' Dr Gibson answered calmly, watching her, looking at nothing in particular but seeing everything.

'Are you even married?'

'No, Mrs Pearce.'

Dr Potter, who was Dr Gibson's assistant, arrived then, and so did the Sister. They came into the office and closed the door and stood beside Marilyn's chair.

'I've decided that the best thing for you would be to have a course of ECT, Mrs Pearce.' Dr Gibson told her.

'What?' Marilyn said in disbelief. She felt a panic begin to burn through her depression, it was as if she had been drunk and had fallen into deep water, suddenly finding that she was drowning and having to strike out desperately.

'A course of ECT, Mrs Pearce. It will bring you out of this depression so that you can go home again.'

'Electric shock treatment? No, I don't want it.'

'Look here, whatever stories you may have heard about ECT, it is quite painless, quite harmless and very effective.'

'I don't want it.'

'All you need to do is sign one of these forms giving your consent.'

'But I don't want to consent.'

Chapter Five: Informed Consent

'Come on now, dear,' the Sister said, 'it will make you feel better again. There's nothing to it. You don't know a thing about it, you're asleep while it's all being done and you don't wake up till after.'

Marilyn began to cry.

'I know you are depressed.' Dr Gibson said sternly but reasonably. 'You may not think you are worth curing—but that is only part of your illness. What about your husband and your child? At least try to get better for their sake! You must be responsible. You can't leave your child without a mother. Don't you owe something to your family at least?'

Marilyn twisted and twisted again at her blouse. It was the same unanswerable argument that she had heard all her life. She was responsible for others, she must do what was right by them, she had no right to cause them suffering. She had never thought that it was so obviously evil to continue to suffer herself. Clearly, she was an even worse person than she had previously believed.

'But I don't want it,' she said weakly, 'I'd rather anything than that.'

'Really, dear,' the Sister said, 'ECT is a very, very good treatment indeed. You'll be feeling as right as nine-pence in a few weeks and you'll be back with your little one.'

'You are here on a voluntary basis.' Dr Gibson said meaningfully. 'Some patients have to be detained against their will. They don't have the same rights as voluntary patients.'

'I think you are letting down your husband and your child, Mrs Pearce.' Dr Potter said slowly, almost as if he was talking in his sleep.

'Really, Marilyn, there's nothing to worry about, it's not nearly as bad as going to the dentist. You don't feel a thing. And in just two or three weeks you'll be fine.' A light-hearted smirk and giggle accompanied the Sister's words.

'Surely you can't want to remain like this for the rest of your life—a sick woman in hospital—while your husband and child fend for themselves.' Dr Potter's words were delivered in the same abstracted, remote tone of someone in the grip of a dream.

In contrast, the Sister persisted with the same invincible cheerfulness.

'I know you're feeling upset and confused, Marilyn dear, but try to be sensible. It's so easy. Dr Gibson wouldn't advise you to have it unless she was sure it would make you well again.'

'Now look here, Mrs Pearce,' Dr Gibson said rapidly, 'I came here today especially to see you. Are you going to tell me I'm just wasting my time? I do have other patients, you know.' Wasting Dr Gibson's time was made to sound like squandering some precious resource, something for which Marilyn might be prosecuted and punished.

Then they were all silent. The three of them said nothing and just watched her. Marilyn swallowed hard and fidgeted in her seat. It was no wonder she suffered — she thought that it was right that someone as evil as herself should suffer. She turned to the Sister who seemed to be the kindest of the three.

'Are you sure it doesn't hurt?'

'It's done when you are under anaesthetic, dear, and you don't know anything about it.'

Marilyn was sitting across the desk from Dr Gibson, who had pushed the ECT consent form right over to Marilyn's side of the desktop. Suddenly, Dr Potter handed Marilyn a pen and she took it unthinkingly and then stared at it in her hand. The three of them were silent again now, and their faces told her that they were resolved not to say anything more unless it was in answer to a direct question from her. Marilyn felt ridiculous as she held the pen, like an absurd child.

Silently, she signed the form.

Chapter Six

The Situation Today

In 2006, when I was approaching the age of fifty, I got to know a young woman in her twenties, seeing her fairly frequently on social occasions, and then losing contact with her in 2009, about a year before I began to write this book. The young woman had a wild, eccentric, extravagant sense of humour similar to my own (some people found it tedious, excessive or 'manic'), but sadly, she also experienced repeated episodes of self-doubt, self-hatred, and despair, which were due to prolonged abuse during childhood, a cause that she recognised perfectly well herself.

Just at the time I lost contact with her, I heard that she had seen a psychiatrist who had convinced her that she was suffering from bipolar affective disorder, which used to be called manic-depressive illness, and I was also told (reliably) that she had been prescribed quetiapine, an atypical antipsychotic drug. Even if the persistent—and increasingly dubious—notion that a distinct, clear-cut psychotic illness called bipolar affective disorder actually exists is true, this young woman showed none of the symptoms described in psychiatric textbooks, some of which have been quoted in earlier chapters.

Her outbursts of wild behaviour were either a natural expression of her personality or they served the purpose of distracting her from her mental anguish, as did her practice of making cuts in her forearms with something sharp. The only genuine therapy for this kind of suffering is reassurance, kindness, support, and a huge amount of effort on the part of the individual herself. Most people consider life to be worth living, but a few people do not believe this, especially in adolescence and early adulthood and in middle age. Those who do not believe that life is worth living often change their minds when they encounter sympathy and understanding from others, or when they pass beyond the two dangerous phases in their development—it is really as simple or as complicated as that.

Quetiapine and all similar drugs merely make an individual's behaviour more acceptable *to other people*, and they expose the individual to the risk of irreversible tardive dyskinesia. Meanwhile, the twin psychiatric and pharmacological industries continue to thrive today. The overwhelming majority of people who complain of anxiety, panic attacks (now called panic disorder), and depression will be prescribed drugs, especially selective serotonin re-uptake inhibitors such as citalopram, escitalopram, and fluoxetine (Prozac), while those who are diagnosed as suffering from severe depression, bipolar affective disorder, or schizophrenia will be given antipsychotic drugs, lithium, and sometimes ECT. Very few people are offered entirely *drug free and non-physical* treatment and support, and other therapies are almost always provided *after* drugs have been prescribed and as an adjunct to them. This overwhelming emphasis and insistence on psychiatric drugs and ECT is confirmed by current psychiatric and pharmacological manuals, including those quoted in this book.

Have things improved, has the assault on liberty diminished? It is certain that many of the practices of the 1940s, 1950s, and 1960s have fallen from favour, and yet the situation today is not a comforting or a hopeful one. A significant insight is given by a textbook designed to teach and train psychiatrists, published in 2008 and still on sale as I write.[1] The book describes a man aged sixty-four who has been 'severely depressed' for several months and has now stopped eating, and although he has been treated with antidepressants, he is suicidal and 'very distressed'. The point of the example is to ask the psychiatrist-in-the-making what treatment would be the most appropriate. The answer is unequivocal: ECT.

---

[1] Cornelius Katona, Claudia Cooper and Mary Robertson, *Psychiatry at a Glance*, 4th edition, Oxford/Chichester, 2008.

Befriending, friendship, companionship, care, kindness, compassion, a little curiosity about *why* the man is in despair, the possibility that he is religious and might be reached through religion, or even the offer of some whisky (perhaps the writers of the book would consider this barbaric and uncertain in its effects) are all quite inappropriate—just ECT. Next patient, please!

The very young are also liable to be treated with quick, convenient, and robust methods, as we see when the writers of the same book remind students that a girl aged sixteen suffering from anorexia can be forcibly fed with a nasogastric tube under the Mental Health Act (usually section 3).

I have commented on the integrity of another (massive) psychiatric textbook in a previous chapter, and in this book we find the disconcerting directness of an account written for psychiatric nurses that would rarely reach the general reader.

> The general picture of acute inpatient wards in England is bleak [...] [T]here is little evidence that inpatient stays are clinically effective or cost-effective [...] providing little more than custodial care [...] Patients admitted on a voluntary basis often experience the admission as coercive, with many subsequently attempting to leave, only to be compulsorily admitted to prevent them from doing so.[2]

The same book also points out, with succinct honesty, that 'the patient group most frequently prescribed ECT are older women who do not have a strong political voice'. The issue of gender is, of course, even more relevant to the situation of psychiatric patients than it is to the loss of liberty elsewhere in society. *Psychiatric and Mental Health Nursing* goes on to present some fascinating reflections on 'post-liberal social control' and the erosion of freedom that has coincided with the September 11 2001 attacks in New York, the bombings in London in July 2005, and the 'War on Terror' generally.

---

[2] Alec Grant, 'Freedom and consent', in *Psychiatric and Mental Health Nursing*, edited by Phil Barker, 2nd edition, London, 2009.

We should be grateful to the authors for pointing out that the 2007 Mental Health Act 'has swung more towards control than liberty'. The 2007 Act adopts a single definition of mental disorder and the term 'appropriate treatment', meaning that 'madness is able to be ascribed by the psychiatric disciplines [...] decisions regarding what constitutes "appropriate treatment" fall to the psychiatric disciplines'. The Act also introduced supervised community treatment (SCT) for patients who have left hospital after being detained there, allowing them to be returned to hospital if they do not comply with the conditions of the SCT.[3]

The political skies have darkened — it is difficult not to think of the 1930s when so much of psychiatric practice was invented — and the outlook for freedom has worsened. (Finally, we should also remind ourselves that Richard P. Bentall stated in *Madness Explained: Psychosis and Human Nature* in 2003 that psychiatric services suffer from a flaw that is 'not one of personnel or resources (although these may be important) but one of *ideas*'.)

A recent study assessed the use of ECT over a period of three months in England in 2006 and compared that period to studies conducted in 1999 and 2002. Specific information on the use of ECT in Britain was routinely collected by the National Health Service until 1991, and then replaced by Hospital Episode Statistics, which considerably underreported the use of this treatment. The authors of the study obtained new information by sending out questionnaires to National Health Trusts. A total of 56 of the 76 trusts that carried out ECT at 109 clinics responded to the survey, and these responses revealed that between January 2006 and the end of March 2006 a total of 986 patients received their first ECT treatment and 899 received a final treatment, amounting to 5,019 applications of ECT. Assuming that the clinics that did not respond to the questionnaire carried out ECT on a similar scale, approximately 1,276 patients

---

[3] Michael Hazelton and Peter Morrall, 'Mental health, the law and human rights', see fn. 2 above.

were subjected to approximately 6,782 applications of ECT in this period of three months. Reading these figures, I have to keep reminding myself that they refer only to England and to a period of just three months.

We have looked at the *experience* of undergoing ECT already, and this is surely the true reality behind the figures. The use of ECT declined between 1999 and 2006, a trend that began in 1985. However, 30% of patients receiving ECT between January and March 2006 were detained compulsorily under the Mental Health Act, and it is reasonable to conclude on the basis of similar studies (see Chapter 1) that the majority of these were made to undergo the treatment against their will — if indeed consent means anything for detained patients, or indeed means very much for voluntary patients. In this book I have argued that consent to ECT is frequently illusory. The number of detained patients subjected to ECT 'significantly increased' between 2002 and 2006.[4] This is, of course, entirely consistent with the culture of 'post-liberal social control'.

ECT is certainly very much still with us, and psychosurgery has not yet disappeared. *Psychiatry at a Glance* (2008), quoted above on the subject of ECT for a man aged sixty-four and forcible feeding for an anorexic girl aged sixteen, tells us that psychosurgery 'is now extremely rare'. About ten operations are performed a year in Britain, usually for severe depression and severe obsessive compulsive disorder, and the techniques have also changed, with anterior capsulotomy and anterior cingulotomy as the favoured methods.

The book states: 'Success rates of 40–60% are reported.' Once again, we should bear in mind Professor Colin Blakemore's words, 'the effectiveness of these operations was evaluated by the very surgeons who had invested their careers in psychosurgery'. In view of the seriousness of surgically destroying part of the brain, we are entitled to wonder if ten operations per

---

[4] David Bickerton *et al.*, 'Trends in the administration of electroconvulsive therapy in England', *The Psychiatrist*, 33: 61–63, The Royal College of Psychiatrists, 2009.

year—well into the twenty-first century—is an encouraging or reassuring figure.

On January 8 2011, a young American called Jared Loughner took a taxi to a shopping centre in Tucson, Arizona, where Gabrielle Giffords, Democrat member of the House of Representatives—by all accounts an unusually decent, humane, and intelligent politician—was meeting her constituents. He calmly paid the taxi driver, and then shot Ms Giffords through the head with a Glock 19 pistol, which had a magazine containing thirty-one bullets. Loughner went on firing, killing six people including Christina Green, a little girl aged nine, and wounding thirteen others before being overpowered by several brave individuals.

In 2010, Arizona had become the third American state—after Vermont and Alaska—to allow citizens to carry concealed guns without a permit. Jared Loughner had bought the pistol he used in the massacre quite legally, and Congresswoman Giffords also owned guns.

The slaughter in Tucson was quickly and degradingly exploited by both Democrat and Republican politicians in the United States, just as the July 2005 bombings in London were exploited—though perhaps less blatantly—by British politicians. Four heavyweight articles by Joe Klein, David Von Drehle, John Cloud, and Michael Grunwald appeared in *Time*, volume 177, number 3, January 24 2011. The killing and wounding in Tucson, the senseless destruction and loss, are undisputed facts, but the *Time* articles—and much else that was written and said about this incident—tell us a great deal about attitudes to mental illness and the times we live in.

Firstly, journalists and commentators felt confident in deciding that Jared Loughner was not only mentally ill, but also in *diagnosing* his illness, and in this respect Joe Klein's article sounds the clearest note of warning. Klein asks: 'have Americans made a grievous error in their policies regarding the confinement of the mentally ill?', going on to tell us that there are 'an estimated 2.4 million schizophrenics in the U.S.', not all violent, but 'a significant minority of them are [violent]'. Mr

Klein does not specify or quantify the 'significant minority', and it is interesting that his article—the first of the four on the subject in the magazine that its readers would come to—elaborates his views on mental illness before even naming Loughner, something that he manages to do only half way through it.

The overwhelming impression given by Mr Klein is that it must be taken for granted that 'schizophrenics' or 'a schizophrenic' killed the innocent people in Tucson. Further, Joe Klein tells us that: 'Until the 1950s, such people [...] were confined to mental hospitals. These were terrible places. [...] It was believed that a new class of tranquilizing drugs could create behavioural miracles.' Of course, he recognises that the miracles did not happen, and he informs us that 'in the 1960s, the streets of most major U.S. cities were teeming with homeless people [...] a significant minority of them mentally ill'. Once again, the 'significant minority' is not given a figure, and it is worth asking if most Americans and visitors to America would recognise the streets of American cities—despite their obvious social problems—in this description of 'teeming' homeless and mentally ill hordes.

Mr Klein adds one significant detail to his description of the sixties, 'At the same time, there was a romanticization of mental illness [in] books and movies like *One Flew Over the Cuckoo's Nest*'. This seems an odd observation to make when writing about the terrible violence in Tucson and its alleged connection with the 1960s. Firstly, the film of Kesey's novel appeared in 1975, and only then was it transformed from a cult book to a widely read bestseller. More important, the novel makes it clear that the patients are too timid to stand up to a tyrannous nurse, and not at all the kind of people to buy a gun or shoot anyone, while McMurphy's violence is confined to fist fights, except for his time as a soldier in the Korean war.

According to Joe Klein, Loughner stated that Kesey's novel was one of his favourite books, joining a list of violent criminals —particularly young ones—who have made similar banal claims about the 'influence' of this or that book or film upon their actions. We might have expected a little more scepticism and a little less naïvety in a journalist of Klein's standing. The close of Klein's article spells out the 'direction' in which he feels that society must proceed: 'reassessing the excessive liberties Americans have granted themselves in recent years.'

The article by David Von Drehle takes Joe Klein's theme several steps further, containing a breathtaking insight into the attitudes of journalist diagnosticians and of psychiatrists also. Drehle states: 'The symptoms and trajectory of his [Loughner's] disease followed the classic pattern so completely that research psychiatrist E. Fuller Torrey could say, without ever meeting Loughner, that "chances are 99% that he has schizophrenia".' It is only rarely that such an enormous — and quite unconscious — example of journalistic gullibility is provided by a journalist, or that such an example of psychiatric dogma is provided by a psychiatrist.

What sane or competent doctor hearing of a young man suffering from severe headaches and fainting — for which there could be dozens of causes — would insist without meeting the young man that the chances 'are 99%' that he has a brain tumour? Psychiatrists, however, feel able to get away with this kind of thing.

In the very same article, Drehle states that Loughner had been drinking heavily, and in the subsequent article by John Cloud it is stated (this was by now widely known) that he had used LSD and other hallucinogens and smoked marijuana excessively. Abuse of any one of these substances can cause paranoid or delusional mental states that may be permanent. A further significant fact also emerges.

Loughner had met Congresswoman Gabrielle Giffords before, at a political meeting in 2007, and asked her this question: 'What is government if words have no meaning?' Drehle regards this question as delusional and nonsensical, but it clearly shows that Loughner had considerable insight into the world we live in, although few politicians — even such a decent and intelligent politician as Gabrielle Giffords — would be prepared to answer it. Ms Giffords did not answer his question, and he apparently felt outraged and bore a grudge against her after that.

Was Jared Loughner mentally ill at the time of the attack? Is there any reason to assume that he was suffering from a psychotic illness? He may have been merely a trivial, inadequate man who was nevertheless capable of a few intelligent insights, so that he felt ignored and undervalued when Gabrielle Giffords deflected his question, and this suggests an instructive parallel. Hitler was just such a mediocre individual, also capable of some penetrating insights, but resentful, jealous, projecting his rage at being dismissed and overlooked onto the society of his day. We know from every responsible history book and every worthwhile piece of research on Hitler that he would have been eminently capable of committing an atrocity like the Tucson massacre if it had suited his purposes. Hitler, however, had organisational skills and huge ambitions that Loughner lacked. The question of whether Hitler and individuals like him are mad or simply evil has been endlessly debated, but no sensible person has suggested that Hitler was a schizophrenic.

Loughner, like other dreary and self-important murderers before him, may have intended to turn the gun upon himself when he had slaughtered enough people to satisfy him, and capture may not have suited his purposes at all. He may also have been quite sophisticated enough to act the part of a 'schizophrenic', only to receive the full cooperation of journalists and psychiatrists with agendas of their own who are willing to diagnose him without even meeting him. Or he may have been permanently deranged by large quantities of alcohol, LSD, and marijuana.

The Republican Sarah Palin was blamed in some quarters for causing Loughner's murderous attack by posting a number of vulnerable Democrat constituencies on her Facebook page with the crosshairs of a rifle marking them, but in fairness this is no more sensible than the diagnoses of psychiatrists who have never met Loughner.

Whatever motivated Loughner, it is clear that his crime is potentially very bad news for human rights and for liberty, and a backlash may be underway. Will the events in Tucson, Arizona, have consequences for the rights of those labelled mentally ill in Britain and the rest of the industrialised world? This is not inevitable, but it is likely in the social and political atmosphere that has prevailed since September 11 2001, which has demonised religious extremists and asylum seekers and led to the extensive use of detention without trial. The old fear of mental illness may become linked in the minds of ordinary people (perhaps deliberately by those with an interest in doing so) with the fear of terrorist attacks.

In 2011 it is clear that the twenty-first century has not started well. The subtitle of Peter R. Breggin's book *Toxic Psychiatry* (1991) is as follows: 'Why Therapy, Empathy, and Love Must Replace the Drugs, Electroshock, and Biochemical Theories of the "New Psychiatry".' We can almost hear the objections of the psychiatric profession as we read these words—yes, all very admirable, but unrealistic, idealistic, and sentimental. However, the opposite is true. Breggin's subtitle sums up the way of realism and hard work, while the promises of psychiatry have turned out to be illusory, unscientific, and profoundly damaging.

Chapter Seven
Freedom, Rights and Rape

Alexander Solzhenitsyn makes one of his many bleakly perceptive remarks in *The Gulag Archipelago*, published in the West in 1974: 'Artificial feeding has much in common with rape [...] The element of rape inheres in the violation of the victim's will: "It's not going to be the way you want it, but the way I want it; lie down and submit." [...] The sensation is one of being morally defiled, of sweetness in the mouth, and a jubilant stomach gratified to the point of delight.' This passage was once again brought to my mind by conversations with family and friends at the time I started to write this book.

My wife and daughter—separately, but in almost the same words—grasped my subject and theme: 'You are going to be writing about violation, about a kind of rape.' Germaine Greer writes about rape with her usual stubborn intellectual integrity and independence (she acknowledges, for instance, that rape is not gender-specific, quoting the Polish anthropologist Bronislaw Malinowski on the rape of men by women), and she confronts the widely held excuse of rapists, that is, the victims enjoy it: 'an orgasm in the course of rape [...] need not necessarily lessen the severity of the trauma [...] if the clear evidence of the victim's sexual excitation makes any difference to his sense of outrage, it is to intensify it.'[1]

---

[1] Germaine Greer, 'Seduction is a four-letter word', *The Madwoman's Underclothes*, London, 1986.

For myself, I found over many years that even my most sympathetic listeners were somewhat sceptical when I likened ECT to rape. I found it striking, therefore, when I came to the following passage in Peter R. Breggin's *Toxic Psychiatry* (1991) describing 'a beautiful young woman lying passively on her back [...] sedated and then rendered limp by the muscle-paralyzing agent [...] Two male physicians and two male orderlies or nurses stand solemnly over her prostrate, vulnerable body. The psychiatrist leans over, places the electrodes on her forehead, and her body quivers as the electricity passes through her brain. The men watch as if spellbound. It is as if I am watching a ritual rape'.

Psychiatric and Mental Health Nursing, to which I have often referred in previous chapters, tells us candidly that ECT 'may exacerbate feelings of shame, failure and badness [...] An apparently successful outcome may simply indicate compliance and powerlessness'. According to this textbook, only a 'minority' feel that they have benefited from ECT.[2]

Depression is lifted by ECT in some people because it disrupts brain function, and frequently damages it permanently, and this happens solely because we need fairly healthy brain function in order to experience depression. However, following the logic of the insights of Solzhenitsyn and Germaine Greer quoted above, the feelings of violation, defilement, trauma, and outrage will be even stronger in many of those patients who have experienced a temporary relief from their depression. They experience the intensified humiliation of the hunger striker who is artificially fed and the rape victim who feels sexual pleasure during violation. To this humiliation is added the desolate and irretrievable sense of loss that goes with having large areas of memory erased.

Sean Haldane, a poet and neuropsychologist, was a candidate for the role of professor of poetry at Oxford in 2010, and in an interview at that time he observed: 'we certainly are not

---

[2] Joy Bray, 'The nurse's role in the administration of electroconvulsive therapy', in *Psychiatric and Mental Health Nursing*, edited by Phil Barker, 2nd edition, London, 2009.

Chapter Seven: *Freedom, Rights and Rape* 125

ourselves without memory. I deal with people whose memory function is patchy. I think it was Bunuel who said "loss of memory is loss of self". From what I observe that is true.'[3] It is fitting that two people who were actually subjected to ECT provide the most eloquent description of its relationship to rape. A registered nurse named Barbara C. Cody stated: 'I call ECT a rape of the soul.'[4] And Melissa Holliday, who appeared in the television series *Baywatch* and modelled for *Playboy*, was no less emphatic: 'I've been through a rape, and electroshock therapy is worse. If you haven't gone through it, I can't explain it.' Ms Holliday's description of how she was undermined by drugs and threatened with being locked up in order to bully her into undergoing ECT proves dismally familiar to readers of Janet Frame, and is no less horrible than the New Zealand writer's experience.[5]

One of the people I talked to when I started work on this book observed that psychiatrists and psychiatric nurses 'believe they are doing the right thing'. This is undoubtedly true, and yet it ignores the capacity that human beings possess that allows them to 'believe' whatever is in their own interests. It has always suited psychiatrists and nurses to believe in the effectiveness of drugs, ECT and psychosurgery—and in their right to force people to undergo these methods—because this belief provides them with a career and a salary. There is also another reason for their conviction.

Peter R. Breggin includes a section called 'Why Would They Do It?' in the chapter on ECT in the book quoted above. In this section he refers to well-documented instances of the 'thinly veiled hatred' that psychiatrists sometimes feel towards patients, manifesting itself in facetious remarks about those they are about to subject to ECT, such as 'Let's give him the works' and 'Hit him with all we've got', or 'Why don't we throw the book at him?' Further, as rape is a crime of anger and an asser-

---

[3] Tim Adams, interview with Sean Haldane, *The Observer*, May 30 2010.
[4] Barbara C. Cody, letter in response to 'Shock Therapy: It's Back', *Washington Post*, September 28 1996.
[5] John Makeig, 'Woman says electric shock treatment destroyed her life', *Houston Chronicle*, June 26 1996.

tion of power, it is often committed against proud, strong, and outspoken women and men, simply because they are more powerful than the rapist. It follows that there would have been a considerable thrill involved in subjecting people like Ernest Hemingway, Janet Frame, and Sylvia Plath to ECT.

If we have blind faith in the authority and expertise of any elite within society, political, medical, or technical, we lose the capacity to think clearly. A blind faith in the self-appointed secular priesthood known as the psychiatric profession may deprive us of the power of clear thinking in more ways than one. Mental illness can be terrifying, both for the sufferer and for those who witness the suffering, and yet the intervention of self-styled experts who use damaging and unscientific methods is no solution at all. There is no clear dividing line between psychotic illness and the inner anguish that we all experience at times. The mental anguish of some individuals is so severe that they need considerable help and support for long periods, or even throughout their entire lives, and this requires a huge effort on the part of society. The methods of psychiatrists are designed to evade making this effort, and they are attractive because they increase the power, prestige, and profits of an elite group.

We need to rid ourselves of the notion that it is acceptable to alter the brains of certain people by chemical, electrical, or surgical means, frequently without their consent or on the basis of very doubtful consent. This notion is not compatible with our present scientific knowledge, and it is not compatible with the conception of human dignity that has developed over the last four centuries. Our attitudes to mental illness need to move forward into the twenty-first century. We need to step forward into the light.